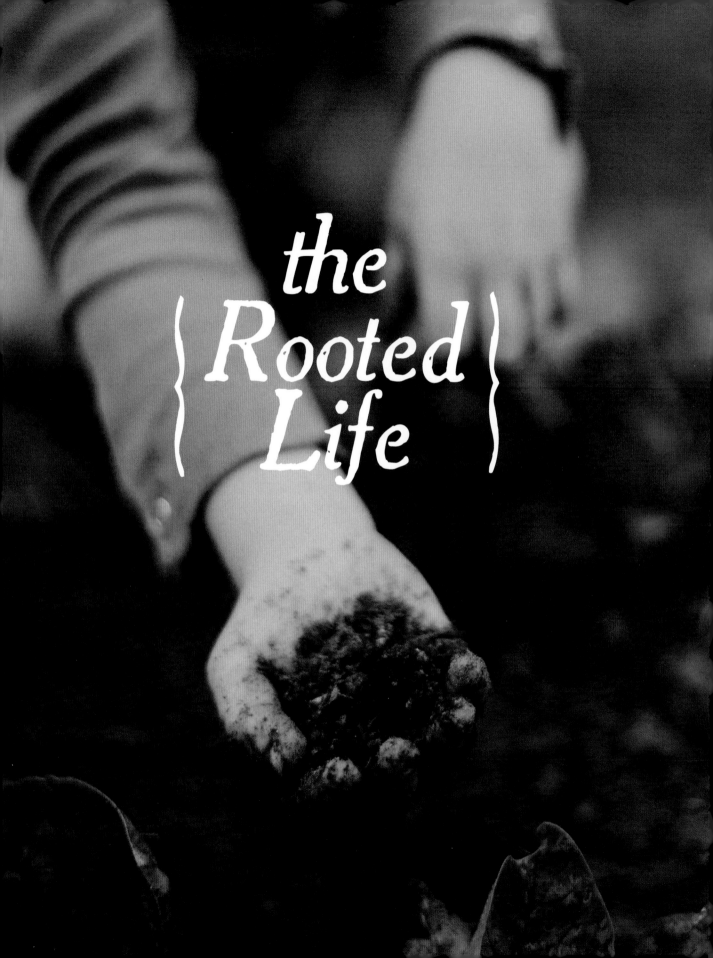

the
{ Rooted }
Life

the {Rooted Life}

CULTIVATING HEALTH & WHOLENESS THROUGH GROWING YOUR OWN FOOD

JUSTIN RHODES

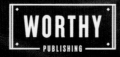

WORTHY
PUBLISHING

New York • Nashville

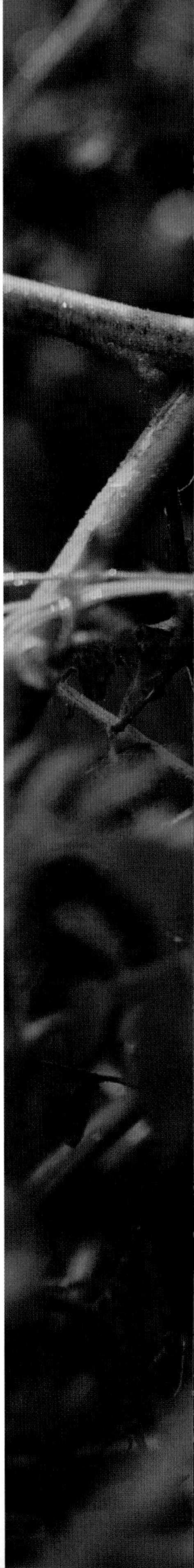

Copyright © 2022 by Abundant Permaculture, LLC

Cover design by Melissa Reagan
Cover photography by Benjamin Roberts

Cover copyright © 2022 by Hachette Book Group, Inc.

Worthy
Hachette Book Group
1290 Avenue of the Americas, New York, NY 10104
worthypublishing.com
twitter.com/worthypub

First Edition: February 2022

Worthy is a division of Hachette Book Group, Inc. The Worthy name and logo are trademarks of Hachette Book Group, Inc.

The publisher is not responsible for websites (or their content) that are not owned by the publisher.

The Hachette Speakers Bureau provides a wide range of authors for speaking events. To find out more, go to www.hachettespeakersbureau.com or call (866) 376-6591.

Photography by Benjamin Roberts

Print book interior design by Bart Dawson

Library of Congress Cataloging-in-Publication Data has been applied for.

ISBNs: 978-1-5460-1259-7 (hardcover); 978-1-5460-1258-0 (ebook)

Printed in China

1010

10 9 8 7 6 5 4 3 2 1

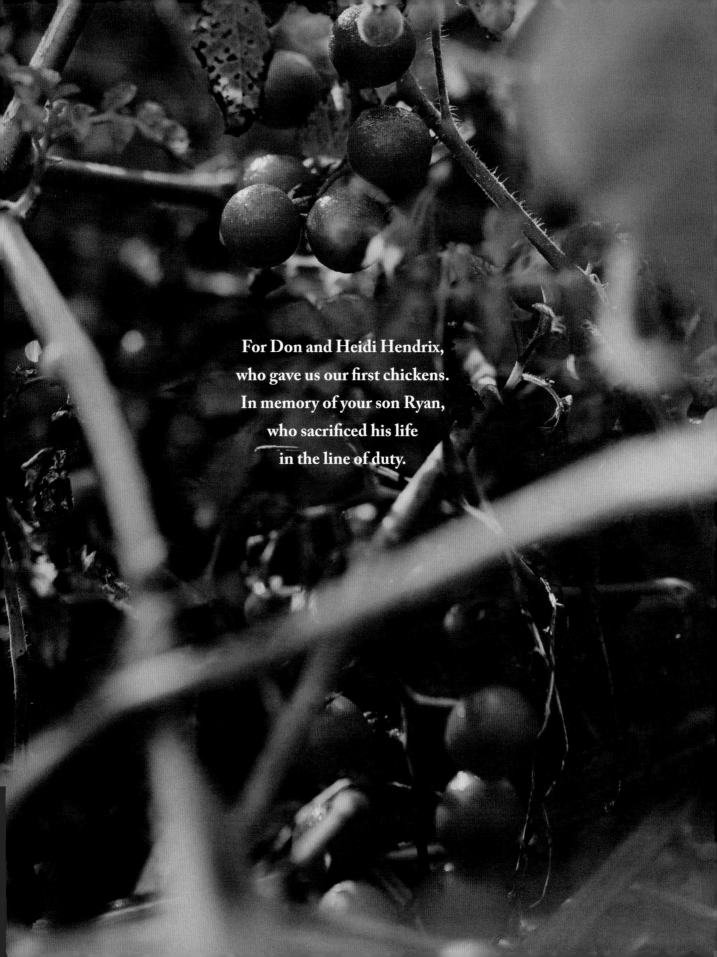

For Don and Heidi Hendrix,
who gave us our first chickens.
In memory of your son Ryan,
who sacrificed his life
in the line of duty.

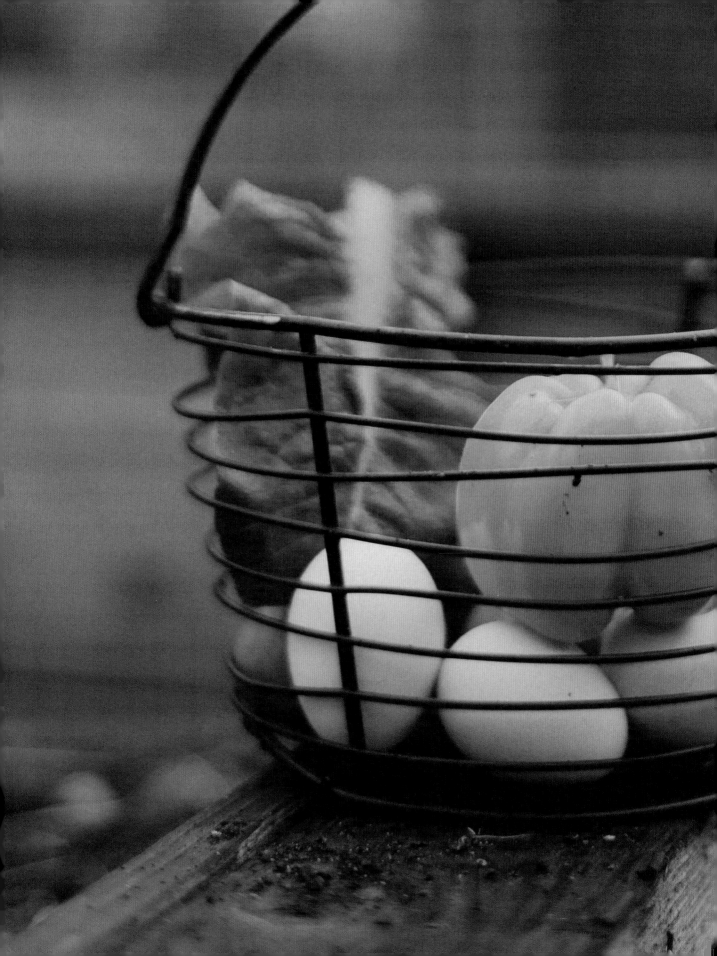

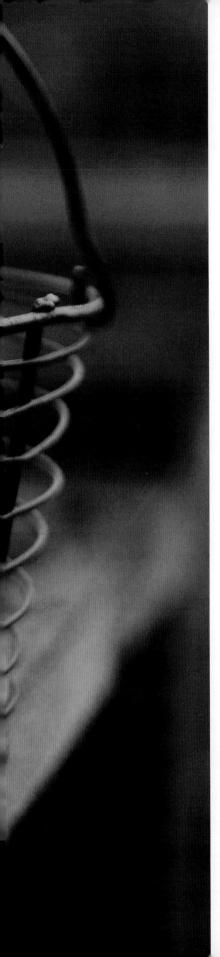

Contents

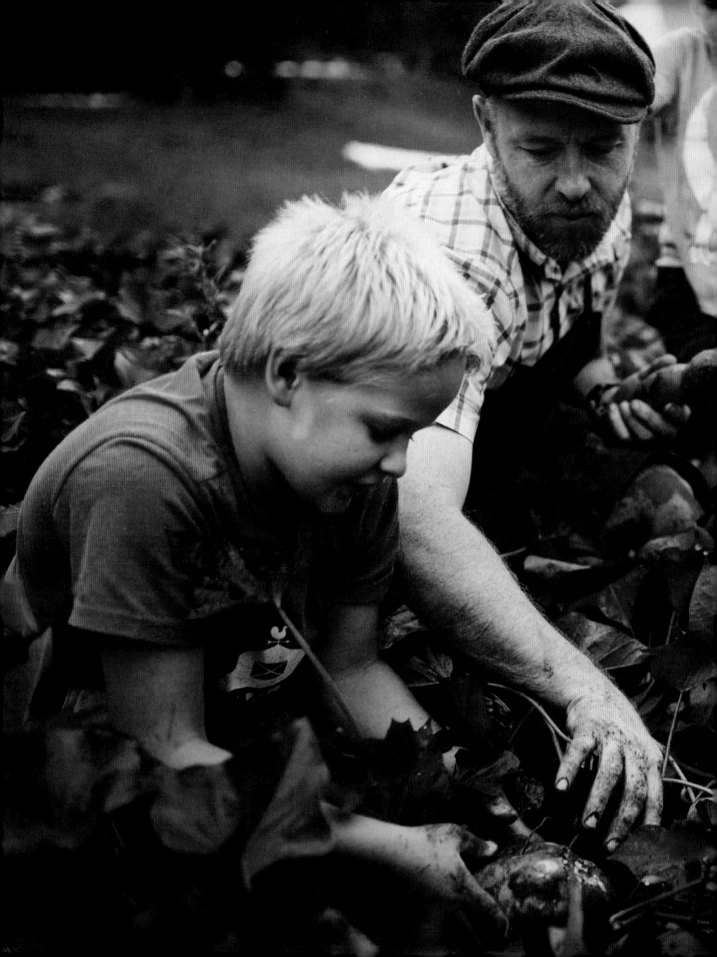

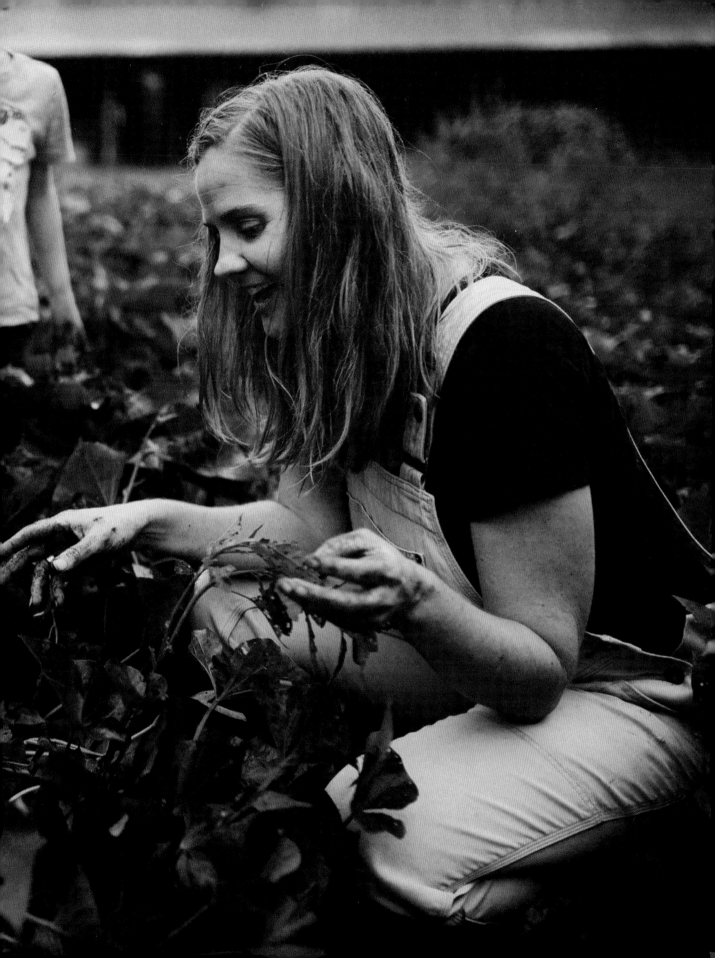

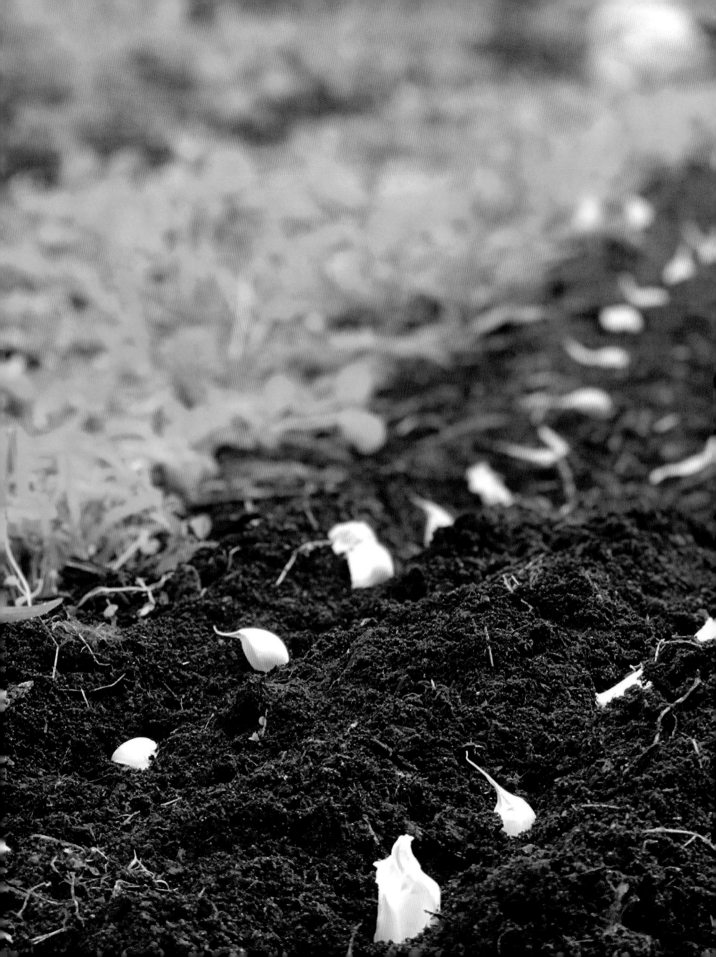

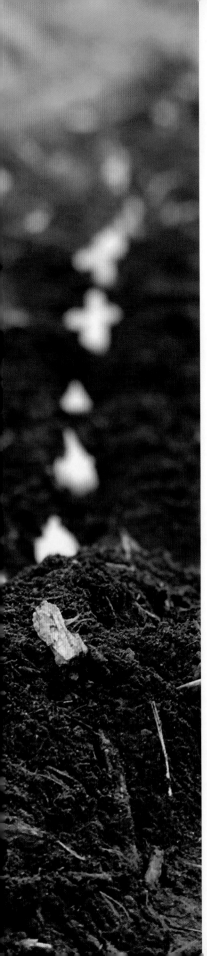

CHAPTER 1

If I Can Homestead, You Can Too

Beep. The cashier slid a bundle of organic lettuce across the price scanner, and I felt my temperature start to rise. Tightwad Justin was getting anxious.

Beep. Another bundle. Then another. I'd never minded being in line at the grocery store before, even when Rebekah and I had our chiddlers (kids) in tow. But now things were different. Now, every time the cashier pulled something out of our still-full cart and beeped it across that scanner, I got closer to a major panic attack.

Beep, my chest squeezed a little tighter. *Beep,* a little tighter still.

It all started a few months before when my wife, Rebekah, read about conventional milk maybe not being great for our family's health—something about hormones or chemicals. I didn't really understand it at the time. She wanted to start buying organic milk instead, and I said okay.

Actually, I said, "Go ahead. No big deal."

Turns out it was a big deal! Because when we ran out of eggs, she started buying organic, free-range eggs instead of eggs in those white Styrofoam cartons I was used to. When we ran out of hamburger, she started buying grass-fed beef. When we ran out of cookies, she started buying Newman-O's instead of Oreos.

We kept going down that rabbit hole until the day I stood glaring at that cashier and wondering how in the world I was ever going to make enough money to feed my family.

Beep. There's the organic whole milk that got us into this mess, $5.99 for half a gallon. *Beep.* Now $8.99 for a box of chicken nuggets with no antibiotics. *Beep.* There goes $7.49 for a loaf of organic bread with sprouted seeds. *Beep.* How in the world can it cost $5.25 for a bag of organic apples? They aren't even Honeycrisps!

Beep. Beep. Beep. My stress level was rising almost as fast as our bank account was falling.

In all seriousness, this was a time in our family history when money was especially tight. Actually, money was nonexistent. Money was credit cards and a prayer for the future. In hindsight, Rebekah was absolutely right about our need for healthy eating—if we hadn't changed our diets, who knows whether one or both of us would still be here today. Even so, the price tag for those changes was sinking us fast.

That's when it happened. I glanced over at the produce aisle and saw a little rack of seed packets. Curious, I walked over and picked out a pack of lettuce seeds. Yes! Just as I suspected, the seeds cost $3, which was right around the same price as each bundle of

organic lettuce the Beautiful One had just picked out.

Reading the information on the back, I started doing some calculations in my head, and—what? Could that be right? This little $3 packet of lettuce seeds would grow literally hundreds of bundles of lettuce if I planted them myself. And if I could harvest seeds from those plants, I could grow hundreds more!

Two thoughts went through my head in that moment. First, why in the world is this grocery store selling seeds? Isn't that counterintuitive? I mean, if people started buying and planting these seeds, they wouldn't need the grocery store anymore! Second, why are there any seeds left? Why haven't people bought them all up? After all, if someone eats twenty-four bundles of lettuce a year, one packet of seeds would last them pretty much forever, give or take a decade. Spend $3 and you've wiped out your lettuce bill for years.

That's really how it started. We bought those lettuce seeds, plus a few other packets. We got some advice from a neighbor who had a garden, and we planted. Then we harvested. And our lives have never been the same.

The Most Unlikely Candidates

I want you to understand from the beginning that Rebekah and I were the most unlikely candidates to jump into the homestead lifestyle. Both of us.

Rebekah grew up in West Palm Beach, Florida, and she spent significant time in swimming pools over three hundred days a year. To this day she can't recall ever getting dirty as a child. Her life consisted of prancing across manicured grass, walking on concrete, and drinking chlorinated water. Those were her points of contact with the earth. No soil involved.

I was a little different because at least I grew up on a farm. Kind of.

My grandfather bought 75 acres of land outside Asheville, North Carolina, way back in 1932. The note was $500, and he paid it off at $25 a month for two years. Fixed up a little house. Started a family. In those days, pretty much everyone had a sustenance homestead of one form or another, and Grandpa was no different. He and his family ate only what they grew—which meant they grew a lot.

My dad always spoke fondly of his

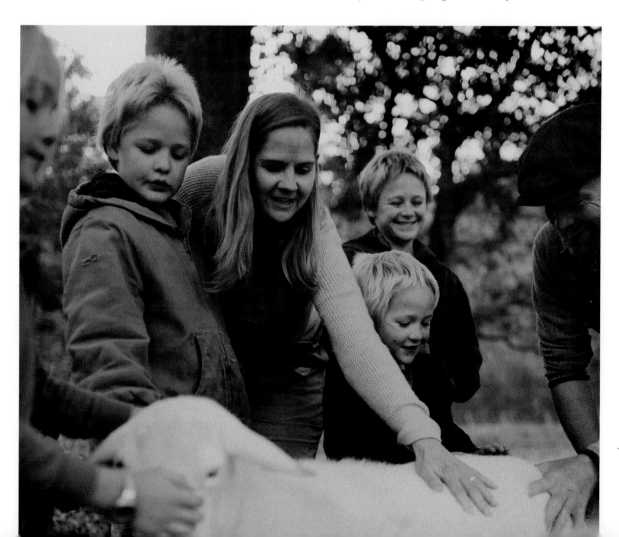

upbringing and the lifestyle of living off the land. Turning the soil. Planting. Harvesting. Running around with animals and learning how to care for them. Pop had lots of fun stories about life on the farm, and he liked to tell them. By the time he grew up, though, Dad was ready for something different. He loved living in the country, and he did keep a few cows when I was a kid, but I think that was mostly for nostalgia. (Also to save money, since you could get a big tax write-off when you used your land for agriculture.)

One time I asked, "Dad, you have such fond memories of growing up on the farm and your parents raising their own food. Why did you stop?"

He just said, "It's cheaper to buy it in the store."

That's what we're all taught these days, right? Growing food is too hard. Growing food takes too much time. Growing food is too labor-intensive. It's much easier to just buy what you need when you need it.

What my dad didn't understand at the time—and what Rebekah and I have only recently discovered—is that the people who tell you that aren't comparing apples to apples. If you want to sustain yourself and your family on processed foods grown from genetically modified seeds, then it really is cheaper to buy that in the store. If you're good with eating meat from cows injected with hormones of every kind and chickens who have never seen

the light of day, it's cheaper to buy that in the store. And if you don't have any problems with pesticides, yes, it's cheaper and easier to buy your fruits and veggies in the store.

But if you're looking for a different kind of life—a life focused on health and wellness—you might need to take a different path. It's really hard to grow mac and cheese. Tomatoes? Not so much. So if you're ready to transition away from sugary cereal and corn chips and toward fresh eggs and fried potatoes, then you need to understand there's no way you'll find that cheaper in the grocery store. That's why Tightwad Justin was about to blow a gasket right there in aisle three!

Here's the good news, though: I've kept track of my own numbers over the years. I know how much I've invested in our homestead, and I know how much we've received as a return on that investment. Here's what I've found:

- If you invest $1,000 in gardens (including all supplies) using the systems described later in this book, you can expect to grow around $2,750 worth of produce at market prices. So, every dollar you invest will return $2.75 in fresh, healthy, organic food.
- If you invest $1,000 in egg-laying chickens, you'll receive about 200 dozen fresh, organic, cage-free eggs in return over the course of five years.

- For every $1 you invest in feed for your meat chickens, you can expect to receive $2 worth of fresh, organic, pasture-raised meat.

All of that brings me back to me. Like I said, Dad was never really interested in farming, and that was especially true once he met my mom. She was from Los Angeles, and she wasn't exactly thrilled to find herself living in a farmhouse in the backwoods of Appalachia. So, we spent a lot of time in town.

I grew up going to school in town. We went to church in town. Most of my friends lived in town. Basically, I was a city boy who happened to sleep and do his homework out in the country. I was encouraged from an early age to go to college, build a career, and buy my food at the grocery store like everyone else.

And that's exactly what happened—until that little packet of seeds planted a dream in my heart of a new kind of life. A rooted life.

The point I'm trying to make here is that neither Rebekah nor I knew what we were doing when we started this journey toward growing our own food. Neither of us inherited the skills, knowledge, or experience to be successful homesteaders. We started from scratch, made mistakes, and learned by doing. And the results have been way beyond our wildest dreams!

The same can be true for you.

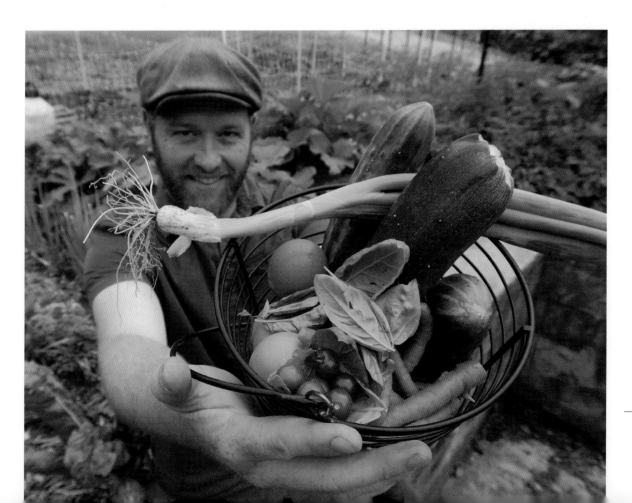

The Case for Growing Your Own Food

Do you remember where you were when you realized you couldn't get toilet paper during the first wave of the COVID-19 pandemic? Of course, for most people the toilet paper thing was a minor issue. A temporary inconvenience. The big story was food.

In 2020, the concept of mass food shortages entered the American vernacular for the first time in generations. There are lots of reasons why that happened, and very few of them had to do with an actual lack of food. Instead, there was a sudden and massive increase in demand as families started buying two months' worth of food instead of two weeks' worth. There were bottlenecks at the processing level. There were supply chain issues.

The long and short of it is that the massive vulnerabilities in our modern food system were exposed, and it happened practically overnight.

Rebekah and I have friends and family members who felt frightened in that moment. Alarmed. Anxious. They went to their local grocery store and found empty shelves. Little or no produce. Little or no meat. The price tags were still in place for beans and flour and other dried foods, but the food itself was long gone. Of course, things got really uncomfortable when people started losing their jobs. Because the only thing more frightening than not being able to find food to buy is knowing you couldn't afford it even if you found it.

Really, it felt like our entire nation and culture were gripped in a kind of panic. There was confusion and chaos as we all asked each other, "Can this really be happening here?"

All of this points to one of the major benefits of growing your own food, which is food security. When you take an active role in cultivating your own food supply, you're less dependent on a food chain that may or may not be stable. This is especially true when you can harvest an overabundance of food at different times of the year and store the excess through freezing, canning, and other types of preservation. (More on that later in the book.)

Basically, growing your own food gives you control over your ability to feed your family. And not just control over the amount of food, but the quality as well. In our experience, the more food you're able to grow, the more control you gain and the more comfortable you feel.

So yes, food security is a huge issue for people around the world today. But there are several other good reasons to pursue a more rooted way of life. For example:

- *Connecting with your food source.* There's a lot of mystery when it comes to the food chain and manufacturing processes out there in the world. What kinds of seeds are being planted? Are they genetically modified? What kinds of pesticides have been used? Are animals being pumped full of growth hormones? Steroids? If a label says "free range," does that really mean free range? How long does food sit on trucks before it gets to the store? How big is the gap between the time food is harvested and the time it actually hits the shelves?

Growing your own food eliminates those questions. It allows you to know what you're eating. It connects you to your food and to the broader story of what makes you tick.

- *Better health.* People are learning more every day about the basic principle that food is medicine. Or the old way of saying it: you are what you eat. People understand that certain types of foods—and certain qualities of foods—will benefit their health. Growing those foods yourself is a great way to ensure they provide exactly what you need.

The reality is you can produce some of the most nutrient-dense foods in the world simply by growing them in your own yard. Why? Because there's a good chance your lawn will have much richer soil than the stripped, exhausted soil of industrialized farms.

- *Saving money.* When it comes to the best foods, the foods that make the biggest difference in the health and wellness of your family, it's not cheaper to buy it at the grocery store. In fact, it's way more economical to grow your own at home.
- *Earning money.* Not only is it cheaper to grow your own healthy food, but you can earn extra money by scaling what you grow and selling the excess. And no, you don't have to make connections with your local Publix or Walmart. I'll share later in the book how to sell what you grow if you're interested.
- *Having fun.* Lots of people grow their own food just to have something positive and fun to do. They like to get outside, they like to be in the sunshine, they like to get a little exercise from Earth's Gym, and so on. Growing your own food can be a positive, productive hobby in the best sense of those words.
- *Taste.* There are many homegrown foods that taste way better than what you can buy at the store. I promise you that's true—not just a little better, but way better! Eggs, tomatoes, strawberries, and carrots are just a few examples.

There are more reasons, of course, but that's a good start. My guess is you already have at least a beginning understanding of why you'd like to grow your own food, given that you're reading this book. So let me offer a little picture—a little taste—of what you can experience when you jump more deeply into the rooted life.

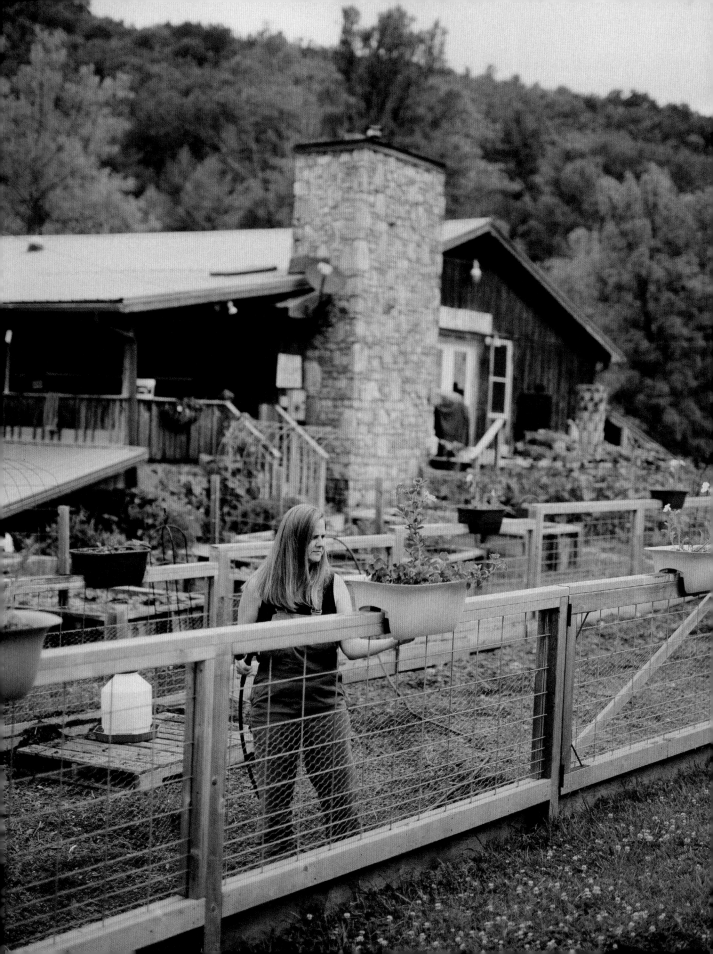

A Picture of the Rooted Life

It was fifteen years ago when Rebekah and I brought home that first packet of lettuce seeds and planted our first garden. Things have changed a lot since then. They've changed for us personally in terms of our mission and purpose, and they've changed physically in terms of our home and what it looks like.

When I walk out my front door, there's a path that leads out to our mailbox at the street. But I rarely notice that path because it's surrounded by gardens. On the left side is our herb garden set in a deep bed of wood chips. We mainly grow culinary herbs there—oregano, dill, peppermint, parsley, cilantro, basil, thyme, sage, chamomile, and rosemary. We pick the herbs at different times of the year, but we cook with them every day. (And yes, when you stand in front of that herb garden, it smells as good as you're imagining right now. Better!)

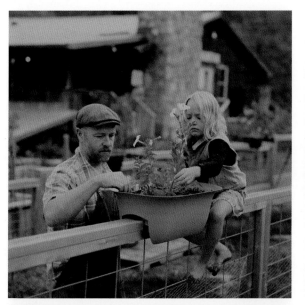
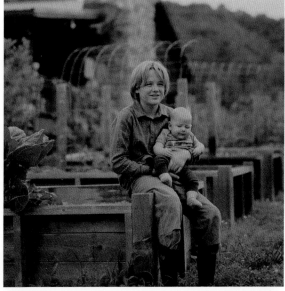
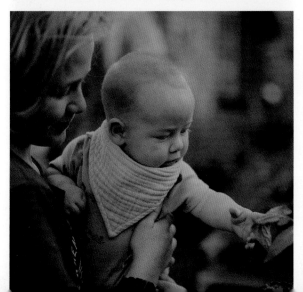
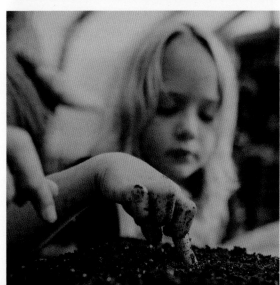

On the right side of the path are six ravishing raised beds that are each packed with growing goodness of every size, shape, color, and texture. The base layer of each container is mostly covered with our leafy veggies—lettuces, spinach, and kale. We've got cabbages and zucchini and green onions. Some of those beds have trellises over the top where the tomatoes can climb. Poking out over all that green are vibrant zinnias, waxy peppers, and several bunches of marigolds to help keep away pests. And I like the way our sunflowers stand above it all like yellow sentinels.

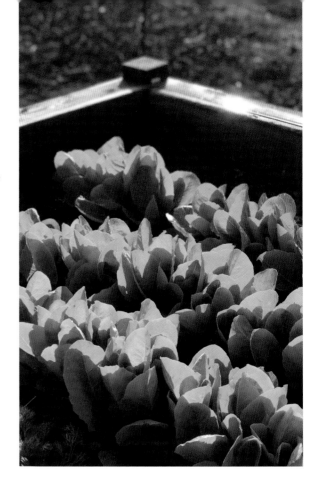

Then, between those raised beds and the street, we've fenced in a permanent enclosure for our egg-laying chickens. If you've never watched chickens before, they are constantly on the move—pecking, scratching, and tilling within the wood chips. It's fun to watch! We also keep a guard goose in that enclosure to stay on patrol against predators.

When I go around the side of the house and walk down the steps, I come to our first greenhouse, which is where we get a lot of our plants and produce started when we grow them from seeds. Then, once things are big enough and healthy enough, we transplant them into the ground in one of our gardens. We also keep asparagus and strawberry gardens right by that greenhouse and close to the water spigot because they give us a place to use that wastewater whenever we wash out our buckets.

All the way at the back of our home is the newest addition to our homestead: a large

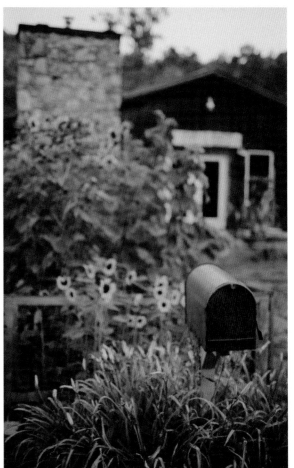

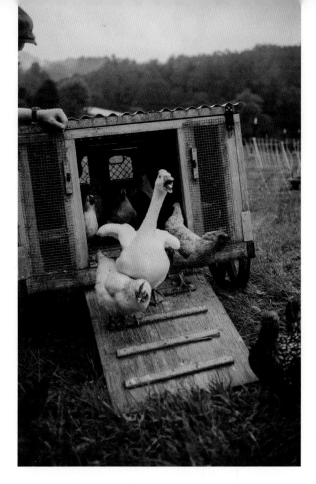

rotate those gardens with heat-loving crops such as cucumbers and tomatoes.

Finally, behind and surrounding all that are the different pastures and paddocks we use for our cows, sheep, pigs, chickens, ducks, turkeys, and more.

Right now you might be thinking, *That sounds like a lot of work!* And it is, although maybe not as much as you think—especially in those big chunks of time between planting and harvesting seasons.

But here's the beauty of it: There are payoffs from this way of life we get to enjoy every single day. Big payoffs. The biggest for me is relationships. I spend the majority of my time with my family each day, which means I spend most of my time with the people I love most. We're in this together—myself, Rebekah, and even the chiddlers from oldest to youngest. We've all been rooted and planted together, and it's beautiful.

pole barn. That's where we house our cows and sheep during the winter, which lets us capture their waste and eventually turn it into compost. Then we've got a separate greenhouse where we keep our egg-laying chickens and our pigs during the winter. The rest of the year those animals rotationally graze around the pastures.

We've installed our Crop Gardens behind that second greenhouse. Those are four 1,200-square-foot gardens that allow us to spread out a little more than the Container Gardens at the front of the house. In the winter, those gardens are packed with lettuces and beets, which means that even during the coldest months, we can harvest fresh salads every day. During the growing seasons we'll

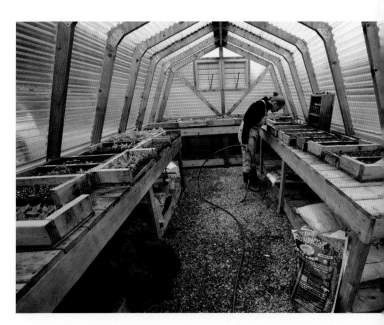

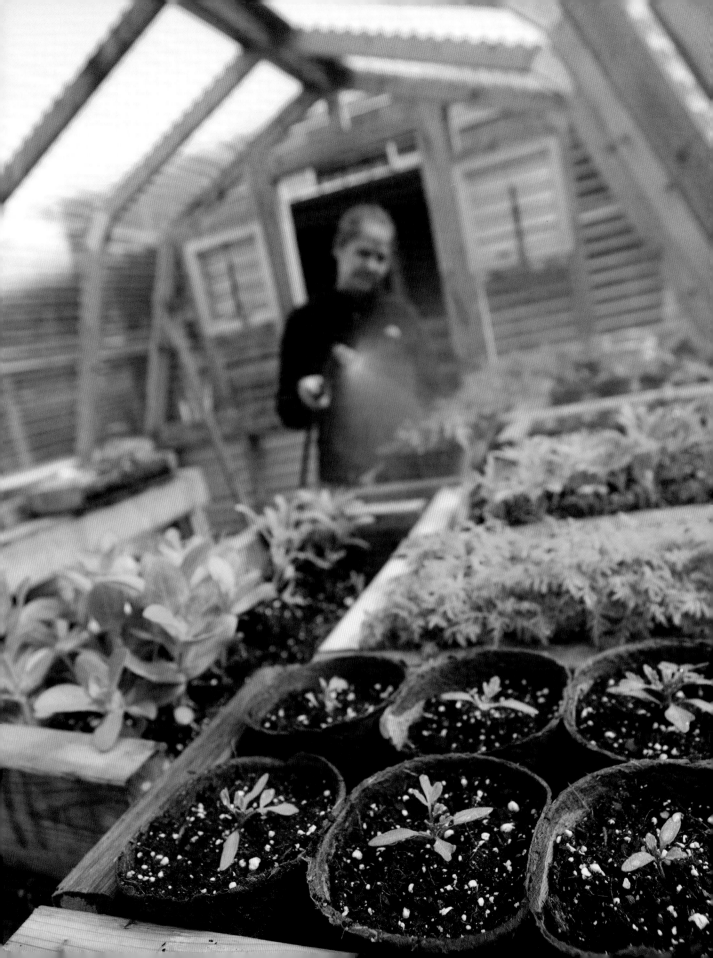

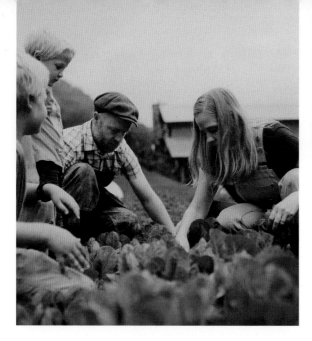
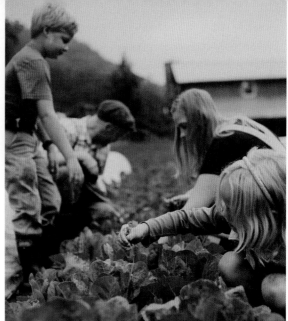

Of course, there are big financial payoffs as well, which Tightwad Justin always appreciates. Depending on the year, we grow 50 to 75 percent of all the food our family eats. We raise all of our own meat, and we harvest the majority of the veggies we eat during the growing seasons. (We do spend some money on produce during the winter, and we've chosen not to grow much to speak of by way of fruit.)

When you boil it all down, we save tens of thousands of dollars every year by growing our own food. We eat healthier than we ever could back in our grocery-shopping days. And we've had many years when we chose to scale up our operation and grow enough extra to sell, which basically meant we fed our family for free.

Now, here's something important to keep in mind: how I live out the rooted life isn't the only way to do it. My family is different from

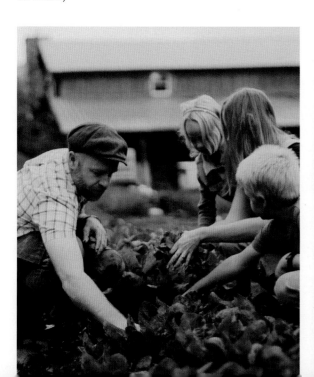
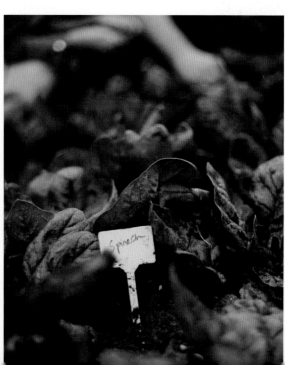

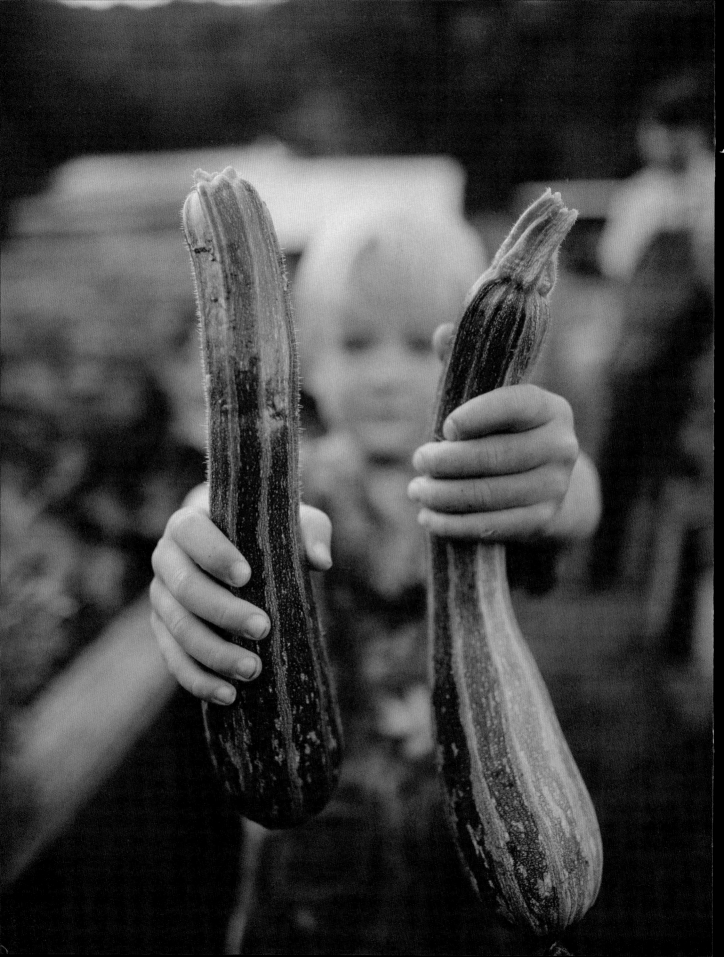

your family, and my situation is different from your situation. So there's no need to do the exact same things we do.

Your rooted life should work for you.

The goal of this book is not to turn you into a full-time farmer or homesteader. Instead, I want to teach you principles and practical ideas that can be applied to most any situation. If you're living in a condo with just a balcony to work with, I'll help you maximize that space to grow as much of your own food as possible. If you're hoping to step up your backyard garden, I can offer lots of ideas and advice. And if you're ready to go the full nine yards and raise chickens along with produce, I'll get you headed in the right direction.

The one thing I can promise is that you will encounter obstacles along the way.

Four Major Obstacles to Overcome

Back near the beginning of our homestead journey, Rebekah and I spent three months in Honduras volunteering at an orphanage. The first day we arrived, I met with the folks in charge and said, "Put me to work. Whatever you want me to do, I'll do."

Well, that might have been a mistake given that the orphanage had 450 kids and only twelve staff members!

Sure enough, they put me in charge of sixty boys living on the property and told me to do three things: One, keep the boys working. Two, make sure nobody runs away. And three, make sure nobody kills anybody else. (That third one was easier said than done since most of my boys were supposed to mow the grass with machetes several times a week.)

The leaders at the orphanage also put me in charge of the farm, although to this day I have no idea why. Rebekah and I had not started our homestead at that point, and I knew next to nothing about farming. Even so, I didn't do a terrible job. In those three months, I managed the egg-laying chickens, and I even cared for about 1,200 meat chickens— raising them from chicks all the way to the harvest.

By the time Rebekah and I returned to our farm in North Carolina, you might say I knew just enough to be dangerous about raising chickens. I was a little naïve about what it would take to set everything up for ourselves. A little overconfident. And that's when we ran headlong into the obstacle I call lack of knowledge.

Lack of Knowledge

To make a long story short, I accidentally killed the first four chickens we owned on our farm. They were egg-layers, and we named them Uno, Dos, Tres, and Quatro after our little jaunt in Honduras. As soon as we got them, we set them up in one of our barn stalls. I was already tasting those fresh eggs.

What I didn't realize at the time was that these young and agile birds were a world apart from the confined meat chickens I'd raised in Honduras. Imagine my surprise when Uno and Dos suddenly fluttered up and stood on top of the stall door, then hopped onto the ground. Wait, chickens can fly?

Yes, chickens *can* fly—enough to get out of a barn stall, anyway. They can also run really fast. I spotted Uno on top of our roof the next morning, but I couldn't catch her. I never saw Dos again. We found the bodies of Tres and Quatro a few weeks later, killed by an unknown predator.

Now that I've got years of experience taking care of chickens, I understand that the birds need to become oriented to a new home before they're set loose. You need to keep them "cooped up" for at least a night. The reason Uno and her posse never came back to our stall was that they were never oriented. They didn't know where home was, so they went in search of one. Simple as that.

I've also learned that while chickens are extremely fast sprinters, they're not distance runners. So if you've got a wayward bird, just keep her in sight by walking or jogging in her direction. Sooner or later she'll get tired out and crouch down in one place. Then you've got her.

So yes, lack of knowledge is a big obstacle for anyone looking to start becoming more rooted or take the next step. Thankfully, this is a relatively easy obstacle to overcome.

The best way to fix a lack of knowledge is to gain it through experience. Just get out there

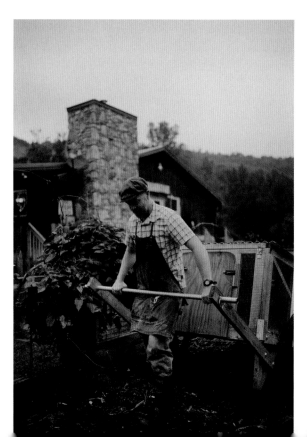

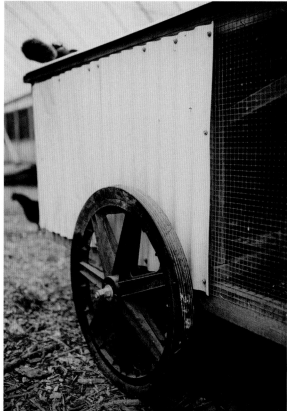

and try. Make mistakes. Learn new things. You'll get the hang of things more quickly than you might think.

Another good way to overcome a lack of knowledge is to seek out know-how from others. For example, Rebekah seems to have a knack for finding just the right author at just the right time. Eliot Coleman. Joel Salatin. Bill Mollison. Each book was helpful in its own way, and each of those authors became a kind of long-distance mentor for our family. (On page 191 you'll find a Resources page with some of the books we have found to be most helpful.)

One of the things I remember about those books is how confident the authors sounded. They spoke with authority. They wrote with certainty. I remember wondering, *Do any of these guys ever make mistakes?*

As you've already seen, you're not going to wonder the same thing about Justin and Rebekah. Not at all. We've made plenty of mistakes, and we're going to be open and honest in sharing those stories with you throughout these pages. That's intentional, by the way. We really hope you can learn something from our failures—just as we did.

In fact, I'd be honored if you think of me as your uncle throughout these pages. That's what I wished for when Rebekah and I were getting started: an uncle who knew what he was doing. Someone I could go see for a brief visit when I had a question or could call up for a quick chat. Someone who could lend a hand and offer some advice so I didn't have to learn everything the hard way.

I've written this book because I'd like to be that uncle for you.

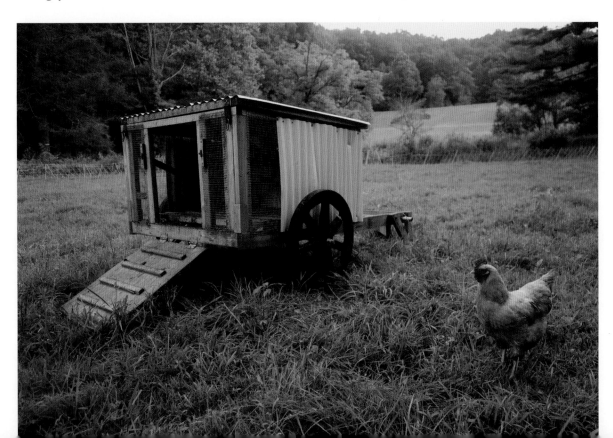

Lack of Money

I mentioned earlier that money was tight for the Rhodes family when we started our homestead. That was a problem because change usually requires resources, and that's definitely true of changing the way you approach food. Growing your own food will require time, of course, but it also demands at least a little financial investment up front.

If money is not an obstacle for you, that's great news. You'll be able to speed up the process. But it's also very possible for people to jump into a more rooted way of life when they don't have extra financial resources—as long as they're willing to be creative and think outside the box.

For example, let me share the two principles that carried our family through those early years when money was a huge obstacle.

Find things that don't cost money. I'm not afraid to admit it: Rebekah and I did a lot of dumpster diving during the first years of our homestead. We were mostly looking for food we could feed our animals, and we found quite a lot of it. But I've also had friends who went through dumpsters at construction sites and found useful building materials for constructing their coops, fences, brooders, and so on.

After a few months, I got a little smarter and started approaching local grocery stores and co-ops. I would introduce myself, talk a little about my homestead and what we were aiming to create there, then ask, "Could I

please have your throwaway produce to feed my animals?"

Many of them said yes. In fact, most were happy to do it, and several local health stores even started setting aside their excess and saving it for me each week. For them, this was a way of keeping food out of landfills and breaking the cycle of waste. There was an environmental benefit for them, and I think they were happy to help someone like me when it didn't really cost them anything.

For me, I was able to feed my chickens for years on 100 percent food scraps, so it was an incredible blessing.

Scale up what you grow. I've always been an entrepreneur, all the way back to my days of selling Saint Bernard puppies as a kid. So when we decided to take things to the next level on our homestead, I knew there had to be a way to pay for the supplies we needed—tools, feed, animals, and so on.

This was right about the time community-supported agriculture (CSA) was becoming popular, and that option immediately clicked with me. So, I hopped on my phone and literally called every person in my contacts over a period of days. "Hey, this is Justin. We've got this homestead, and we're starting to grow a little more. Thinking about selling some. Would you be interested in eggs, chicken, or produce?"

Turns out people were interested. It was a great deal for our customers because they could get healthy food at a cheaper price than

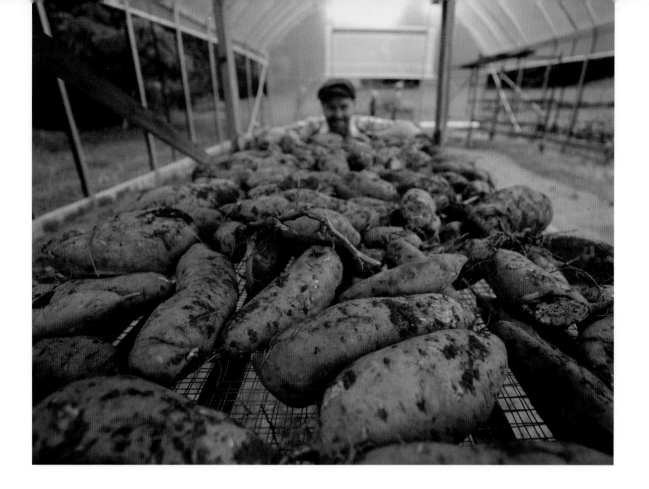

the stores, and they knew it was raised well. It was a great deal for Tightwad Justin because our customers paid up front each month, which meant I could actually afford to buy feed and supplies. Best of all, the money from our customers paid for the food our family kept in addition to what we sold. So, we ate for free.

The basic idea here is that it doesn't take much more to grow four raised gardens instead of two. It doesn't take much more to raise twelve chickens instead of six. And it doesn't take much more to raise two cows instead of one. So, scale up what you plan to grow, sell the extra, and keep what your family needs at no cost to you. You may even have some money left over to buy your spouse something nice.

Lack of Energy

As someone who has dealt with chronic Lyme disease for years, I understand energy isn't a resource all people can take for granted. There are limits to what we can give. When it comes to a rooted life, lack of energy can be an obstacle for many reasons—if you're a senior, for example, if you've got an illness or disability, or even if you've got a family and a career and you're trying to squeeze growing your own food into a schedule that's already packed full.

For those situations and more, let me offer three pieces of advice on how to pursue a more rooted life in spite of a lack of energy.

Make your plans ahead of time. Geoff Lawton, one of my first homesteading mentors,

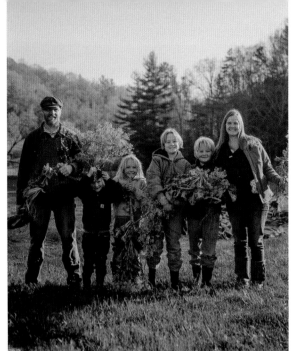

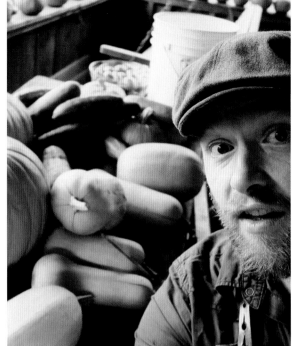

told me, "It's easier to make mistakes on paper than in real life." I have found that to be true over and over again. So, one of the best ways to deal with a lack of energy is to plan out what you want to do before you start doing it—and then review that plan a few times to look for problems or weaknesses.

Now, if you're young and full of vigor, I really do recommend you get out there in the ground and just plant. Try things. Make mistakes. Have fun! But if energy is an obstacle, planning first will help. In Chapters 2 and 3 I'm going to walk you through practical steps for making a plan and designing

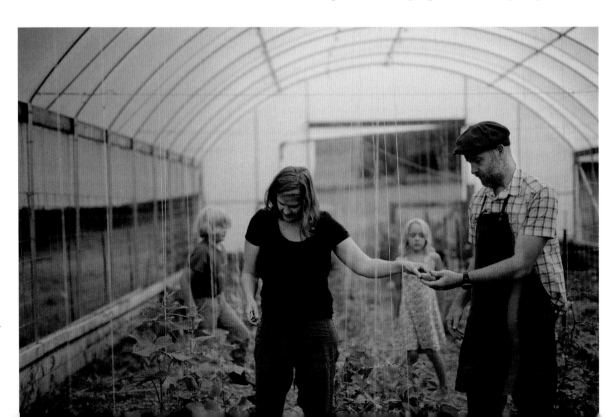

your growing system in a way that works best for you.

Do what you can. When people start growing their own food, one common mistake they often make is trying to do too much. Seems like everybody wants to do everything. So a good way to combat a lack of energy is to resist the temptation to do everything that pops into your brain. If all you can manage right now is growing a pot of basil to put on your pizza, start there. Move on when you're ready.

Once again, I'm going to be your uncle Justin here. In the next chapter, I'll show you how to start smart with growing your own food, prioritize those projects that are most important, and let go (for now) of those ideas that don't really make sense for where you are now.

Tap into your community. Finally, a great way to overcome a lack of energy is to tap into the energy of others. Rebekah and I still do this all the time. We'll ask people to help out with bigger projects like butchering chickens or filling raised beds. Most of the time people are happy to say yes. Why? Because they are eager to learn. They want to be more connected to their food story, which makes them very willing to help.

So, who can you ask for help? Is there someone who might enjoy spending a couple of hours with you each week as you weed the garden or plant some seeds? Is there a neighborhood kid with a strong back who might enjoy earning a little money by spreading compost?

Here's the truth: When you bring people into the process of growing food and reconnecting with the land, you're helping them as much as they are helping you. Maybe more. And I say that from experience.

Lack of Vision

One of the biggest obstacles that can hold you back from anything you want to achieve—including a more rooted style of life—is what I call a "scarcity mindset." This is really a worldview defined by lack. It's the idea that there's not enough out there. Not enough resources. Not enough money. Not enough time. Not enough talent.

You'll know you're dealing with a scarcity mindset if you use two words often: *never* and *can't.* "I'll never have . . ." "I can't see how . . ." "I could never . . ." "I can't do that." Your focus is consistently on the reasons why your goals or your dreams are out of reach, and will always be out of reach.

In other words, a scarcity mindset is based on fear—that plus a lack of vision for what could be.

Let me shoot plain with you: such a mindset is death for the rooted life. That's because the rooted life is all about abundance.

One thing I would encourage you to do right now, right here at the beginning of your journey toward a more rooted way of life, is to think deeply about what I call an "abundance mindset." Put simply, that's the opposite of a scarcity mentality. Abundance says there is enough. Nature has enough to go around, but, more importantly, you have enough within you to achieve your dreams—enough resources, enough talent, enough time, enough intelligence, enough motivation. You have more than enough!

An abundance mindset says that your goals are there for the taking. If you put in the hard work and take a chance, your dreams are within reach—including your dream of growing your own food and moving your family to a more rooted way of life.

The point I'm trying to make here is that you will encounter obstacles when you start growing your own food, and especially if you jump more fully into the rooted life and everything it represents. But those obstacles can be overcome! That's the great news, and that's what I'm going to help you do throughout these pages.

You Are the Hero of This Story

Our earliest homestead dreams were filled with juicy cabbages, lush landscapes decorated with frolicking chickens, and a family laughing and working together while each of us enjoyed our glory day in the hot sun. That's what we thought the rooted life would be like.

What actually happened? Cabbages so devoured by bugs we had to peel off the first ten layers before we could find anything to eat. Chickens free-ranging and pooping on our sidewalks and scratching the mulch away from our trees. Losing our prized rooster, losing four out of our first five sheep, and having to turn our precious family cow into hamburger because of her failure to thrive. What also happened was a family happy to work together most of the time but with kids still quick to quarrel and abandon their assigned jobs.

So yes, we left out the struggles when we first dreamed about homesteading. But here we are with reality all around us, and we haven't given up. That prompts the question: What keeps us here? What makes it worthwhile?

Believe it or not, a big part of the answer to those questions is the struggle we face each day.

Have you noticed that every epic movie has a character who wants something? They have a goal. A dream. A quest. In the end, they either reach that goal or not. (Usually they do get there because we all like happy endings.) But if that's all there was to it, the story would stink. It would be boring. Problem identified and problem solved.

Instead, what happens in the middle of those movies? Struggle. Striving. Stress. There are all kinds of obstacles that stand in the way of our hero, and they must be overcome.

Well, guess what—you are the hero in this

story! You want to take control of your food. You want to know where it comes from. You want healthy, affordable nutrition for yourself, your family, and your community. But you don't exactly know how to make all that happen. You're not sure how to get started.

That's why I'm here to help you out. I'll be your Gandalf, and this book is your map. Seriously, all you have to do is read and do. Learn and practice. Keep that up, and you will have a happy ending. Countless homegrown meals for you, your friends, and your family.

Looking back on my own story, it's true that dreamy visions of our own private Utopia first got us excited about growing our own food—but we've stuck around for a surprisingly different reason. We've found joy in our calloused hands. We take pride in the blood, sweat, and tears required to get that fresh food on our plates. That's what makes serving it and eating it so sweet!

We sit down to a meal together and we say, "We grew this." We remember the stories. How we picked up our baby chicks at the post office early that first morning. How we protected these green beans from weeds and bugs. Oh, and don't get me started on the ice cream— milking all those tiny cow teats and moving the herd to new grass. Every. Single. Day.

Our family swells with pride because we were actually part of the struggle. Part of the story. We remember starting that lettuce in the greenhouse, transplanting it, picking off the yellow leaves, watering it, weeding it, and finally harvesting it with the chiddlers. Those potatoes. We remember sticking the seed potatoes in the ground without letting them scab over (not recommended) to see if it would fly (it did). We remember moving those meat chickens to new grass every day and making sure their fence was always electrified so they'd be protected from predators.

It's a joyful, proud feeling to say the least. We set out to grow healthy food for our family, and we've arrived! And we didn't get here because we're unicorns without any problems. After all, we're farming real animals and plants while working with wild and unpredictable nature. Yes, it's *hard*. But that's exactly what makes it so special.

Now I get the chance to take what we've learned and lead you on your own food-growing adventure. The great news is I've already made most of the mistakes, so you don't have to.

Let's do this!

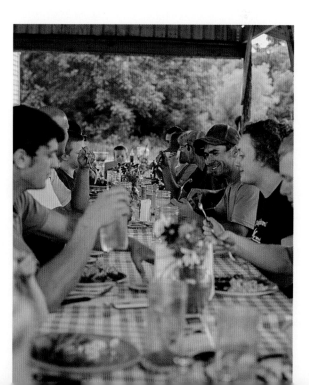

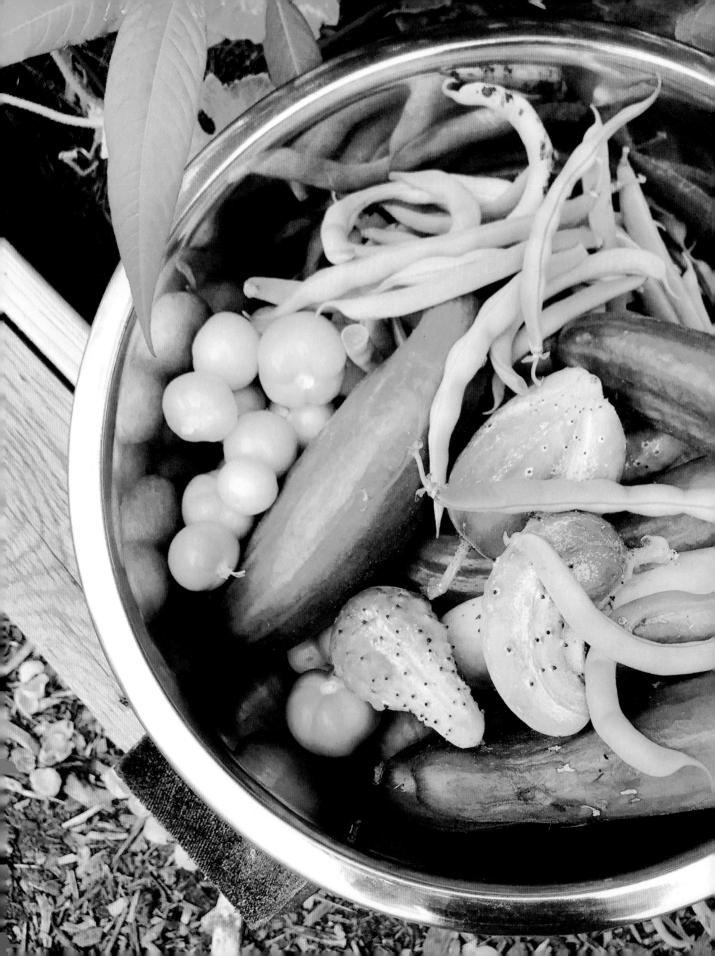

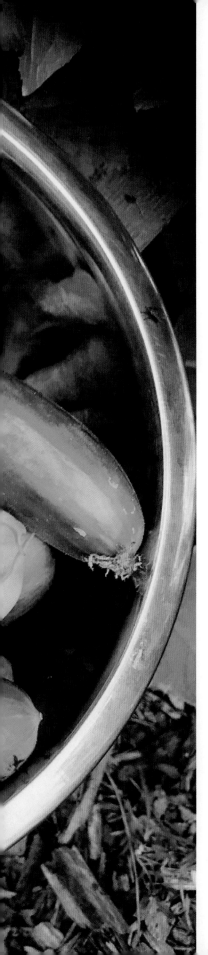

CHAPTER 2

Starting Smart

"Justin!"

She yelled so loud I could hear her voice over the loud clatter of my string trimmer, and I froze. After being married for five years to my high school sweetheart, I knew by her tone and volume. I was in deep doo-doo.

This was Saturday morning. All week we'd been planning to work on our overly ambitious first garden during the weekend. It was getting late in the growing season, and we were tired from balancing multiple priorities. But we wanted to finish strong. We were committed.

As each day ticked by, I kept thinking I should try to get a little done here or there so our workload wouldn't be ridiculous on Sunday—but I had other stuff to do. It was a busy season. "I'll get to it tomorrow" became my mantra.

Sometimes the Beautiful One asked me how the garden was looking, and I'd walk over to the window and squint against the sun to try to see what was growing 130 feet away over in a corner of the backyard. Everything seemed okay. "Looks like there might be a few weeds coming up," I'd call out over my shoulder. "Nothing major."

Well, Saturday finally came. I decided to earn a few husband points by going out early and putting in some sweat before Rebekah showed up. But as I approached the garden, panic rose in my chest. Weeds that had looked minuscule from the bedroom window were actually quite daunting. They were completely overrunning whole patches of the garden, including an area off to the side where Rebekah had planted some prized peppers.

Thoughts whizzed through my brain. *I've got to do something fast! All week I've been telling her it's all good down here, but it's an absolute mess!*

Then it hit me: our string trimmer. I could fire it up and string-trim the garden to knock out those weeds in minutes instead of hours. What a brilliant idea! This could actually revolutionize the way we garden and even the way others fight back weeds. It seemed so wonderful and attainable I wondered why no one had ever thought of it before.

Everything went splendidly. The weeds were blasted away, and I reveled in wielding the power of my machine. Just as I was about to finish—taking a moment or two to admire my work, of course—I heard Rebekah scream. I heard my name. And then I heard the question that froze me to the bone.

"Where are my peppers?!"

I looked up at her agonized face. I looked over to the spot where her peppers were growing—or *had been* growing. I looked down at the string trimmer still humming in my hands.

I knew.

Rebekah stormed off in order to preserve her religion. I chased after her. Lamely. "At least we can still buy peppers at the store!"

"I don't want store-bought peppers." Her voice was flat. "I wanted our homegrown peppers because they taste so much better."

She was right. You simply can't buy that kind of quality at the grocery store. Rebekah forgave me, but she never forgot. To this day she'll tease me about mowing down her prized peppers.

I learned two valuable lessons that day. First, string trimmers have no place in my garden. Sure, I might use them to cut some grass clippings *for* the garden but never *in* the garden. Second, I realized I needed to place that garden a lot closer to our house.

The truth is Rebekah and I chose a horrible place to start growing our own food. And I mean physically horrible. Like many well-meaning but clueless food adventurers, we haphazardly picked out different spots for the different elements of our homestead, and then we just kept adding on new things in new spots without any kind of a plan.

Gardens? Let's put them out back where we've got that flat patch by the woods. Chickens? We've got an empty stall in the barn downstairs, so the chickens can fit in there. Strawberries? They would probably look pretty out here in the side yard. And on and on.

Remember what I said about sharing our failures? Setting up our different elements this way was a big mistake! I want to help you avoid making that same mistake, so we're going to walk through five basic rules that will allow you not only to start growing your own food, but to start smart.

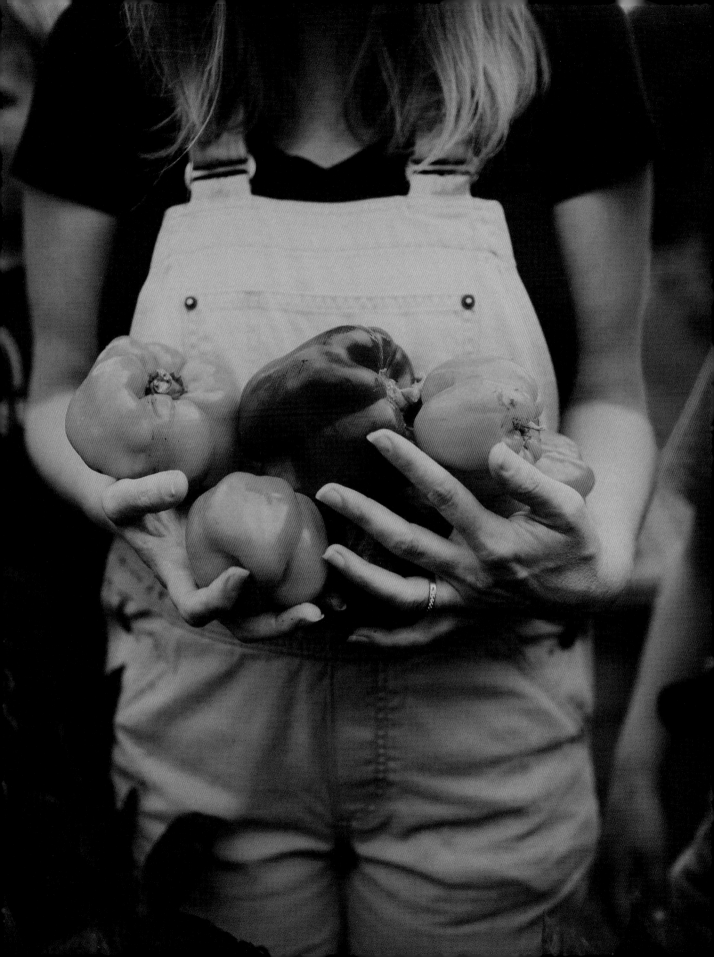

Rule 1:
Start Right Outside Your Door

Yes, I mean this literally. When you're ready to begin growing your own food, the best place to start is right outside your front door.

Why? Because when you place your gardens or other elements right outside your front door, you're going to interact with those elements every time you leave the house and every time you come home. You're going to walk by what you're growing several times a day. That way you see the weeds. You see the tomatoes ripe for harvest. You see what needs to be done, and you're already right there to do it. No need to walk sixty-three steps each way.

The problem Rebekah and I encountered was that placing gardens and other growing elements far away from the house made them easy to ignore. It made them easy to neglect. "Out of sight, out of mind" is a reality.

Thankfully, after more years than I care to admit of trudging that 130 feet between our gardens and our home—plus zigzagging around to other areas—we finally got smarter and moved the majority of our operation to the front yard. We have only a seventh of an acre there, but we've packed it full with six raised beds, a chicken run, a thriving herb garden, a medium-size Crop Garden, a couple of small berry patches, and two fruit trees.

Not only does our front yard look fantastic because of all that growth and life, but it's convenient. It's so much easier to manage!

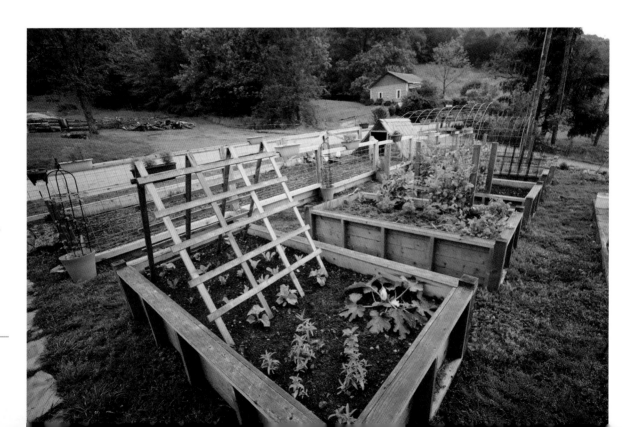

What about you? When you walk out your front door, what do you see? I'm willing to bet that whatever you find there has primo potential to be a food-growing paradise.

But maybe all you have outside your front door is a balcony and then an asphalt parking lot, because you're in an apartment or condo. That's okay! Balconies and porches are great places to start a Container Garden. You choose the type of container based on the space available, you fill it with potting soil, and boom! You're ready to grow just about any culinary herb you can think of. But don't stop there. Container gardens are also great for leafy greens like lettuces or Swiss chard. You can grow tomatoes, peppers, and even potatoes if your container is deep enough. (More on how to do all that in Chapter 3.)

In short, even with just a small porch or balcony, you can still supplement your nutritional needs every day with healthy versions of your favorite foods.

Now, if you've got even a little yard at the front of your house, the options get much wider. You can still do Container Gardens, but they will look more like raised beds, and you'll have more room to spread out. You can expand your herb garden and still grow those leafy greens, tomatoes, peppers, and so on. But now you can add sprawling plants like pumpkins and squashes. Or, when you build directly on the ground for what I call a Bulletproof Garden, you can grow everything I already mentioned, plus corn and beans and other crops.

Growing in your front yard also makes it possible to install some mobile chicken systems or even a permanent coop and chicken run. That gives you both meat and eggs, and lots of them!

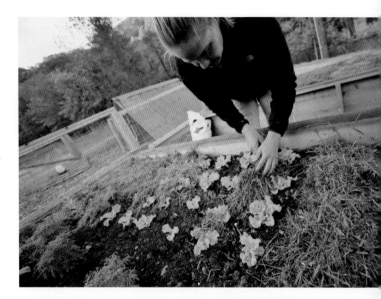

Of course, if you've got a lot of space on your property, then your options are basically unlimited. You can plant Crop Gardens and grow all your produce at a much higher scale. You can raise cows or sheep or turkeys and keep them rotating on just a few acres. You can even plant fruit or nut trees.

My point is this: whatever you identify as your main goals for growing your own food, don't overcomplicate things at the beginning. Start right outside your front door.

Rule 2:
Start Outside the Door of Your Heart

There's a funny thing that often happens when people decide to grow their own food for the first time: They get delusional. By that I mean they decide to grow things they've never eaten or don't really enjoy.

People who are new to the rooted life can get roped into fads, or they can get too caught up in the idea of being as healthy as humanly possible. "Look at how much kale we can grow!" Well, that's great news if you're really into kale. But if you're more of a meat-and-potatoes kind of family, there's a good chance most of that kale will go to waste.

That's what I mean when I talk about starting outside the door of your heart. Start by understanding what's most important to you, and then grow what you enjoy most.

If you're a meat-and-potatoes kind of family, for example, grow meat and potatoes! If you like to eat big salads every day, grow what you need for those salads. If you have a hundred favorite recipes that are all based on eggs, get some egg-laying chickens and harvest as many of those little protein miracles as you can.

The critical thing here is to understand why you want to grow your own food. Is it food security? Is it health? Are you trying to earn money? Those factors should be the primary influence on how you set up your food-growing system and what you choose to grow.

Now, here's a tip. The Bible says, "Where your treasure is, there your heart will be also." So, one of the best ways to determine where your heart is focused is to check your money. Specifically, check your grocery store receipts. What foods are you spending the most money on each month? What food does your family like most? What food makes you most excited?

That's what you should grow.

Of course, if you spend thousands of dollars on Doritos and Froot Loops and Coca-Cola, you're going to have a hard time growing that. So you need to continually go back and evaluate why you are interested in the rooted life in the first place. But as a general principle, you'll have the most success if you start by growing what you enjoy most.

Rule 3:
Start Small

I don't know exactly how it happened, but one year Rebekah and I let our spaghetti squash planting get out of control. That particular crop is easy to grow and it stores well, so we planted an entire 24 x 50-foot Crop Garden with nothing but spaghetti squash. We went spaghetti squash berserk!

I still remember when harvest came and we spent most of the morning wheelbarrowing—yes, I said wheelbarrowing—loads of spaghetti squash from the garden to the house for storage. Man, we were excited! We felt like we were swimming in spaghetti squash.

Then came the meals. Spaghetti squash at lunch. Spaghetti squash for dinner. If you haven't tried it, reheated spaghetti squash isn't as good as it sounds. It's a little squishy. After just a couple of weeks, our whole family pretty much decided we didn't like spaghetti squash anymore. In fact, it's a good thing our pigs *love* spaghetti squash, because we were over it.

The next year we decided we'd be fine with

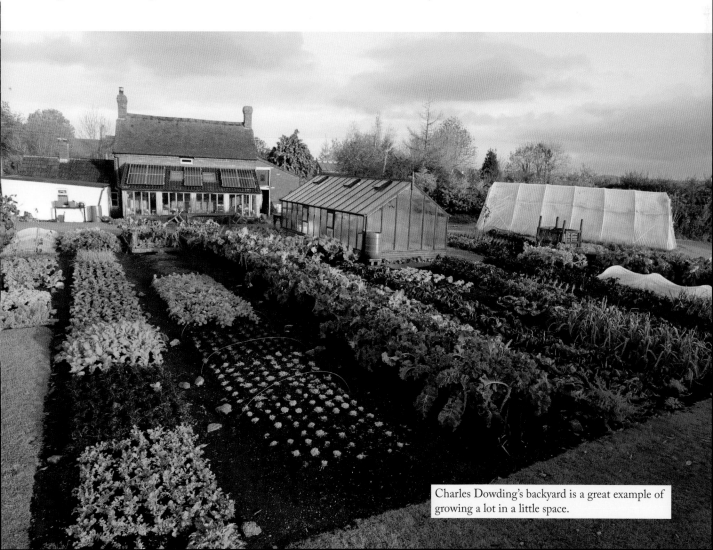

Charles Dowding's backyard is a great example of growing a lot in a little space.

just one or two squashes a month for half the year. You can get that with just a couple of plants. Maybe four at most. So, we were a little more realistic in our planting that season.

Here's the moral of my story: it's best to start small when you begin growing your own food.

I've seen a lot of people get caught up in grandiose visions and dreams about their version of the rooted life. "When I get this property or when I finally have this much time, here's what I'm going to do." Realistically, though, how are you going to manage a 5-acre dream homestead if you're not maxing out the small backyard you have now? Truth is, you aren't.

It's much better to start small and work your way up than to start big and immediately feel overwhelmed. Fortunately, you don't need a whole lot of space to grow a whole lot of food, which is something Charles Dowding has proven many times over on his farms in the United Kingdom. Just look how much bounty is possible in a small garden plot! It's productive, it's beautiful, and because he dedicates all his energies into that small space, it likely returns way more than he needs.

Benefits to Starting Small

Here are a few quick benefits you can enjoy when you choose to start small and prioritize what matters most for your specific needs.

Minimize failure. You'll fail smaller when you start small. And that's important because

you are going to fail. That's guaranteed. But there's a big difference between killing a 20-acre bumper crop of hemp and finding a few cabbages that got eaten to smithereens by bugs.

It's better to fail small, count your losses, and learn from your mistakes.

Hand tools. Going small means using hand tools and small machines rather than investing a ton of money in something industrial. I'm talking about scythes and reel mowers for mowing a lawn, plus hoes, pitchforks, wheelbarrows, and a minivan.

Yes, I said minivan. Sorry, guys, but you don't need a truck for the rooted life. I farmed for years with a minivan. To this day I don't have a truck. I borrow one if needed, but I have found a Suburban with a trailer to be the ultimate "bring the family along" farm vehicle.

Save time. Starting small also means you won't have to invest as much time in your endeavor. Again, you really don't need that much time, work, or space to grow a significant amount of your own food.

How much time will you need? Here's a quick breakdown:

- One family working five hours or less a week gardening and keeping laying chickens in a small yard can grow up to 50 percent of their own food during the growing season.
- One family working ten hours a week gardening, keeping laying chickens, and

raising meat chickens on less than half an acre can easily grow 50 to 75 percent of their own food during the growing season.

- One family working twenty hours a week on 2 to 5 acres can grow over 75 percent of their own food year-round.

To get a better understanding of the different options available to you, and how much time each of those options will require, check out the Best Homestead Elements chart at the back of this book (page 193).

The 1 Percent Rule

Here's a quick tip for when you do start digging in on the actual work of growing your own food: you can make tremendous improvements and accomplish huge things by just changing 1 percent every day.

For example, if you have a big project you want to tackle but you don't have the time to make it happen, the worst thing you can do is wait until that magical moment when you suddenly do have enough time. Why? Because that magical moment will never arrive. It's a mirage.

Instead, take tiny steps. What I call

1 percent changes. You don't have ten hours free to tackle that big project today, but can you start by doing something for six minutes? That's 1 percent of ten hours. Maybe tomorrow you can dedicate seven minutes. Then eight. Then ten. Eat the elephant one bite at a time.

Right now there are countless things I need and want to do on the farm: improve my winter cow/sheep pole barn, install underground water lines, create more pasture, build a cover over my chicken run, build a shed, set up a permanent butchering station, and the list goes on. Obviously, there's no way I can have it all finished today. Actually, I've been in this long enough to realize I'll never arrive. There will always be something else that needs to get done. So, I just take steps forward—even if they're baby steps—and my soul is mostly satisfied.

It's like when my kids get a new Lego set to build. They become so frantic to get it finished! I have to remind them, "Hey, slow down. Isn't building the fun part? Enjoy the process."

Well, I should heed my own advice. "Slow down, Justin. Enjoy the process. After all, the journey *is* the destination."

Rule 4:
Make a Plan

I've never built a house from scratch, but I have managed several construction projects here on our homestead. For each one, we sat down and put together a plan on paper before we bought supplies and started cutting wood. That just makes sense, right? Nobody puts up something as important as a building without first developing a strategy for how to get it done.

Well, the same should be true when you build your food-growing system. So, let's finish this chapter by working through five quick steps that will help you plan out a functional, convenient system for growing your own food in your own space.

Step 1: Write Out Your Goals

The first step in making your plan is to write out all the hopes and dreams you have for your food-growing adventure. And I do mean all of them! If you've ever considered having emus or alpacas or Sasquatch or devil's eyes (what I call goats), this is the time to put those dreams in ink.

Remember what Geoff Lawton says: "It's easier to make mistakes on paper than in real life."

For example, you might be really interested in growing specific types of foods:

- *Vegetables:* lettuces, kale, Swiss chard, asparagus, celery, tomatoes, peppers, potatoes, cabbages, onions, garlic, squashes, pumpkins
- *Fruits:* apples, peaches, pears, grapes, cherries, berries, bananas, avocados, melons, citrus, figs, dates, tropical fruits
- *Herbs:* oregano, dill, spearmint, peppermint, parsley, chives, cilantro, basil, thyme, sage, fennel, chamomile, lavender, rosemary, wheatgrass
- *Nuts and seeds:* peanuts, almonds, cashews, pecans, walnuts, sunflower seeds
- *Producing animals:* cows, goats, sheep, chickens
- *Meat animals:* cows, pigs, turkeys, chickens, ducks

Those are all great options, and it's always good to know what you want. However, another way I encourage people to think about goals is to determine how much of your own food you want to grow in a specific time. For example:

- I want to grow enough produce to have fresh salads for lunch once a week.
- I want to grow 25 percent of my family's produce needs (fruits and veggies) for half the year.
- I want to grow 50 percent of my family's total food (vegetables, fruits, meat, and dairy) during the growing season.

MY TOP 5 FOOD GOALS

What do I want to accomplish?	When do I want to accomplish it?	Priorities 1–4 (see Step 3 on page 39)

- I want to raise 75 percent of my family's meat and 50 percent of our produce during the year.
- I want to grow 90 percent of our family's total food for the year.

Another way to approach one or more of your goals is to think in financial terms:

- I want to save $100 a month by growing my own food.
- I want to cut back our monthly food budget by 25 percent.
- I want to cut back our annual food budget by 75 percent.
- I want to earn $100 a month by growing food that I can sell.
- I want to fully support our family's finances by growing enough food for us to eat and selling the extra to replace my salary.

Now it's your turn! What are your goals? What are your dreams? Remember, this is a great time to be specific, but it's the wrong time to think about practical stuff. Don't worry about details or what's realistic. This is a brainstorm, and it needs to be a safe place to dream.

Step 2: Identify Your Parameters

Okay, now it's time to get practical. I know, I know—it's much more fun to dream, but we've got to buckle down eventually. So, the next step in planning out your food-growing system is to identify your parameters. Meaning, you need to be open with yourself about both your opportunities and your limitations.

Here are some of the main restrictions you'll need to consider as you determine the food-growing system that works best for you.

Time. Each of us has only twenty-four hours every day, and all of us have to sleep. So, you need to determine how much time you can realistically invest in growing your own food. If you and your spouse both have careers and commute to the office, for example, that will severely restrict your opportunities for working your system. On the other hand, if you spend a significant amount of time at home, you will be able to do much more.

Here's the good news: most families will be able to grow at least 50 percent of their own food during the growing season if they invest just ten hours a week. That means one hour a day on weekdays, and then half a day on the weekend. Ten hours right there! Or thirty minutes on weekdays and a full day on the weekend (or two half days). One of my favorite recommendations to "find" the time is to cancel your fitness club membership and spend that time in Earth's Gym.

Physical space. You can't grow property, so another key restriction is the amount of space you have available for your food-growing system. If you really want to raise cows for meat and milk, for example, but you're living on a 5,000-square-foot plot of land in the

MY PARAMETERS

How much time can I invest each week in growing my own food?	
How much space do I have available?	
What can I grow based on my climate zone?	
What are my windows for growing seasons?	

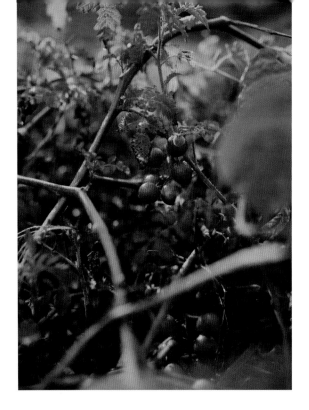

middle of the suburbs, you will probably need to set that dream aside. For now.

As I said earlier, though, you don't need a huge amount of space to grow an abundant amount of food. If you have a quarter acre, you've got more than enough space to grow 50 to 75 percent of your family's produce needs, and you can also raise chickens to supplement meat and eggs. That's an incredible amount of food! And it will be incredibly good, I promise.

So, how much space do you have available for growing your own food? Go ahead and take a walk around your home to identify your options, opportunities, and limitations. And remember: start right outside your front door.

One more thought: if space is at a premium for you, there may be an opportunity to expand a little by accessing a community

garden. These have become more popular in recent years, and you can grow quite a lot even in a little patch of earth.

Climate. Where you are in the world does have a big influence on what you can grow. Let's say you have a dream of growing mangoes and other tropical fruit, but you live in Connecticut where the temperature goes below freezing quite often. In that case, it really will be cheaper (and easier) to buy your tropical fruit at the grocery store.

You do need to honestly assess what you can grow in your specific climate. Fortunately, much of that work has already been done for you. Just go to Burpee.com to find your growing zone and see exactly what will thrive in your space.

Energy. The final major restriction is the amount of physical energy and labor you are able to invest in growing your own food. Of course, if you're young and full of energy, this isn't really a restriction at all. Get out there and plant!

But if you do need to think realistically about your energy reserves, or if you are working through an illness or a disability of some kind, then take a moment to honestly assess yourself. How much of your energy can you commit to this more rooted way of life?

Remember, we're already starting small. So don't let this be an obstacle that prevents you from getting started.

Step 3: Prioritize

Once you've got a big list of your dreams and an awareness of your restrictions, it's time for the rubber to hit the road as you prioritize what you plan to tackle first.

Take out your big list of dreams and label each one with a number between 1 and 4. Labeling a goal as "1" means it's one of your top priorities. A "2" means this is something you'd like to add to your food-growing system in a year or so. A "3" is more of a longer-term plan. And "4" means, *What was I thinking? This is ridiculous!*

Keep in mind two big questions as you work through your list of dreams. First, *What is most important?* And second, *What is realistic?*

Are you ready? Go ahead and start marking those 1s, 4s, and everything in between.

Speaking of 4s, don't take out a Sharpie and cross out those wilder dreams. That's not what I'm suggesting here. The idea is that you're not giving up on those hopes or goals, you're just going to come back to them later.

Step 4: Study

But not too much. Don't get caught up in analysis paralysis. You will *never* learn everything. Heck, I'm still learning on a weekly basis by texting my friends, making mistakes, and researching online.

So, take a little time to study up on those key priorities in your list. Get a general idea of what it's going to take to make them happen.

What is your climate zone? What supplies are you going to need? Are you in the right season to start growing, or do you need to wait until it gets a little warmer?

One time we thought about breeding our own guard geese to keep watch over our chickens. But after a little chat with Mr. Google Pants, we found out it takes geese a long time to bond with each other—and there's a chance they won't ever bond. After that research, we decided it wasn't worth the effort and we'd just keep buying geese instead of breeding our own. That's how study can help.

If you're looking for some places to start, we've listed many of our favorite books, websites, and more on the Resources page at the back of this book (page 191).

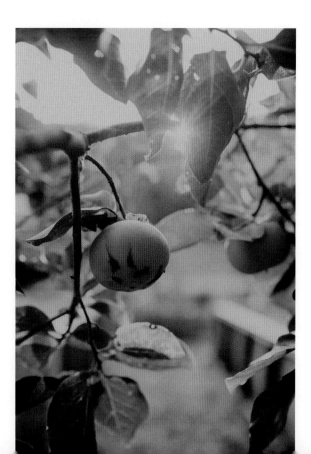

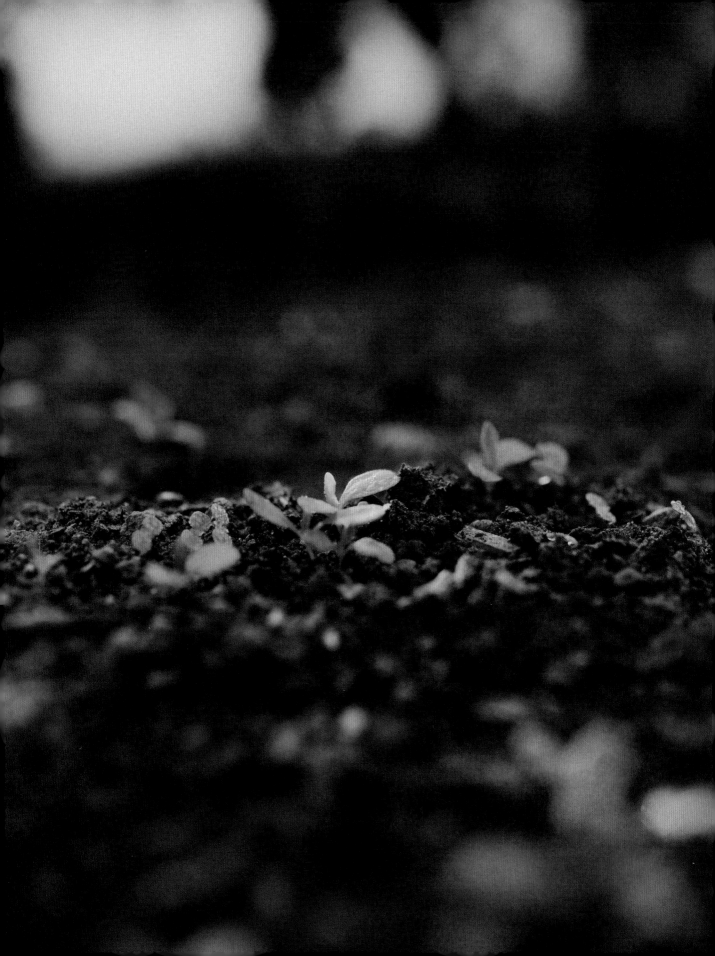

Step 5: Work and Rework the Plan

The most important thing you can do to learn how to grow your own food is to get out there and do it! And that's what Step 5 is all about. Once you've got your priorities and you have a plan for what you want to grow and how you're going to grow it, the next step is to make it happen.

In other words, close this book and get started! (Although maybe don't close it quite yet. You probably want to learn a little more about smart design, gardening basics, harvesting, chicken ninja stunts, and getting your family into the rooted life. But then, once you've read through those chapters, put the book down and get started!)

Not only do you need to work your plan, but you need to rework that plan periodically as well. By that I mean it's important to evaluate what's going well, what's not going well, and how you can tweak your food-growing system to be as productive as possible.

For example, I already told you about the hassle Rebekah and I went through for years because our gardens were placed too far away from our front door. That was our original plan, but it wasn't the best plan. So, we fixed it.

You'll go through the same process, which is great news. Why? Because that means you're learning.

One more thing: you are going to fail. That's nothing personal, it just happens. To all of us. You may water your asparagus too little, or bugs might get your cabbages. Sometimes

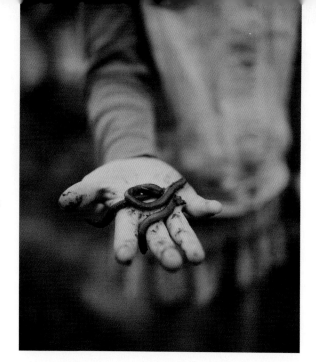

these obstacles will be defeating. Sometimes they'll be devastating. You might even lose whole crops. Things might get frozen or never flower in the first place.

Say it with me: "It happens. It's okay."

Also, you may have heard the saying, "Where you have livestock, you'll have deadstock." Take it to heart because it's true. Something is going to die. Most of the time it won't be your fault, but sometimes it will be. Just remember that every failure, mishap, mistake, and obstacle is actually an opportunity in disguise.

I like that moment in Anthony Doerr's book *All the Light We Cannot See* when von Rumpel wonders, "What did his father used to say? See obstacles as opportunities. . . . See obstacles as inspirations."

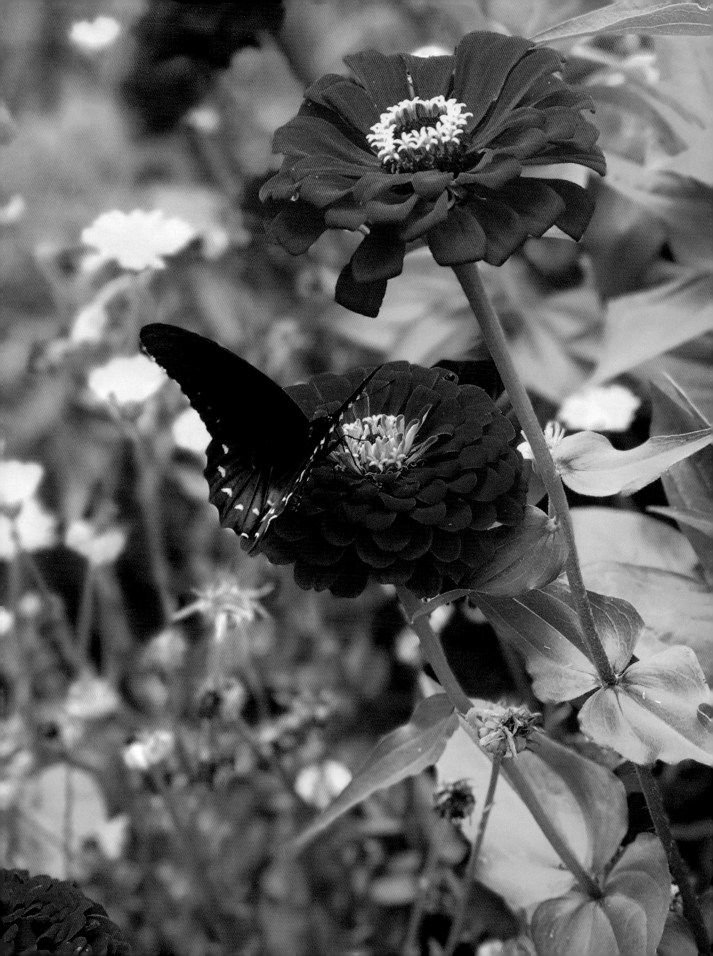

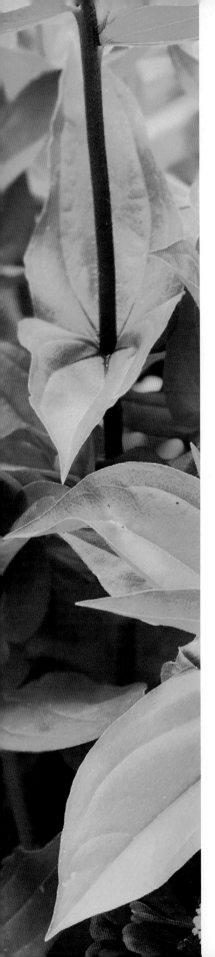

CHAPTER 3

Gardening Basics

We called it the Great American Farm Tour, and it was one of the most interesting and exciting experiences of our lives. Also exhausting. And terrifying. But lots of fun.

This was in 2017, when both the Beautiful One and I were feeling some angst about our homestead and our place in the world. You know how if you grow up in a specific religion there comes a moment when you need to make it your own? That's what we were experiencing with our farm. We didn't feel as rooted as we thought we should.

So, we uprooted ourselves for ten months to visit farms and homesteads in every state across America. (Yes, including Alaska and Hawaii.) We sold all our livestock, shut down our gardens, bought a bus, converted it into an RV, and hit the road—chiddlers and all. Our goal was to both showcase and learn from the different ways people grow their own food all around the country. Somewhat secretly, we were also exploring whether we could find someplace better to set up a homestead.

To make a long story short, we found a lot more on our tour than farms and homesteads. We found the America you don't see on the news or in the media—happy, content, helpful, and collaborative. We visited with people of every race, ethnicity, and creed, and without exception, everyone was generous, offering us hospitality and, in some cases, even opening up their own homes to us.

It was beautiful.

It was also educational. We met with farmers who grew their own food in Minnesota, where it gets down to –60°F in the winter. We met with folks growing gardens and raising goats in Arizona on just 3 inches of rain a year.

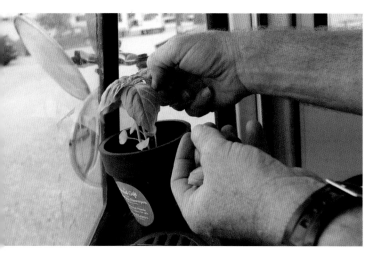

And when we got back to our own place in Fletcher, North Carolina, we found something especially sweet: a home. We realized we were in the best place in America for us, and we became more rooted to our farm and our land and our lives than ever before.

Here's a little detail you might enjoy. In the middle of our trip, we picked up a packet of basil seeds in Iowa, along with a little 4-inch pot and some soil. This was July. We planted those seeds and set up the pot next to our windshield so it could get enough sun. (We had to buy a Velcro patch at Walmart to keep it in place.) By mid-August we were in Wyoming, and we were harvesting leaves from our Bus Basil to go with our pizza!

Now, that food had a story!

You know what I call that? Gardening. Growing your own food. And that's exactly what I want to show you how to do in this chapter. Specifically, we're going to explore three types of gardens that will help you cultivate health and wellness by growing a significant portion of what your family eats every day.

No matter where you are or how much time you can invest in the process, you can use one of these three methods to get stuff growing. So let's plant!

The No-Excuses Container Garden

The first gardening system I want to show you is what I call the No-Excuses Container Garden. And that's really what it's all about: no excuses. Doesn't matter where you live, doesn't matter what kind of soil you have, doesn't matter what weather you deal with—you can grow your own food in a Container Garden.

One of the people we visited on the Great American Farm Tour was our friend Ken Randall (@IslandHomesteader). He lives on an island in the Outer Banks of North Carolina, which means he doesn't really have soil. He's got sand and rocks. Plus, his home was built on top of an old parking lot, which means his "yard" is compact and impenetrable.

Still, Ken grows an incredible amount of food through his Container Gardens. He even grows potatoes, for crying out loud! (That's a big deal because they require a lot of soil.)

What is a Container Garden? Just what it sounds like: instead of growing fruits and veggies in the ground, you grow them in containers. You can place these containers just about anywhere—on a balcony or deck, on your windowsill, in your kitchen, in your yard, on the dashboard of a bus, or all of the above.

What kind of containers can you use in a Container Garden? All kinds! That includes:

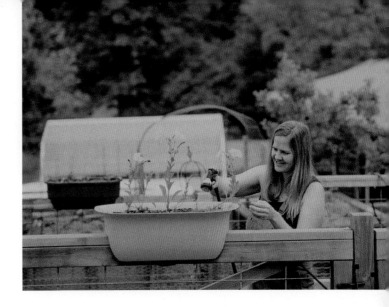

- *Terra-cotta pots:* These are naturally beautiful and low cost. Just be sure to keep your plants watered, because these pots can wick away moisture.
- *Wooden containers:* Build your own pots or boxes out of wood, convert something, or purchase new. Just make sure the wood isn't pressure treated and has openings in the bottom for water drainage.
- *Hanging baskets:* These are a great way to make use of vertical space. Be sure to water them thoroughly and fairly often.
- *Fabric pots:* They can range from beautifully designed small pots on

Wayfair all the way to mega growing areas from Gorilla Pots.

- *Pretty much anything:* Old boots, bathtubs, toilets, buckets, and many other objects can be recycled into gardening containers. Ron Finley, aka the "Gangster Gardener" in south-central Los Angeles, is famous for using old dresser drawers as growing containers. Whatever you choose to use, just make sure your containers are made of nontoxic materials and have drainage at the bottom.

What can you grow in a Container Garden? Probably more than you realize:

- *Herbs:* oregano, dill, spearmint, peppermint, parsley, chives, cilantro, basil, thyme, sage, fennel, chamomile, lavender, rosemary, wheatgrass
- *Leafy greens:* lettuces, kale, Swiss chard, broccoli, cabbages

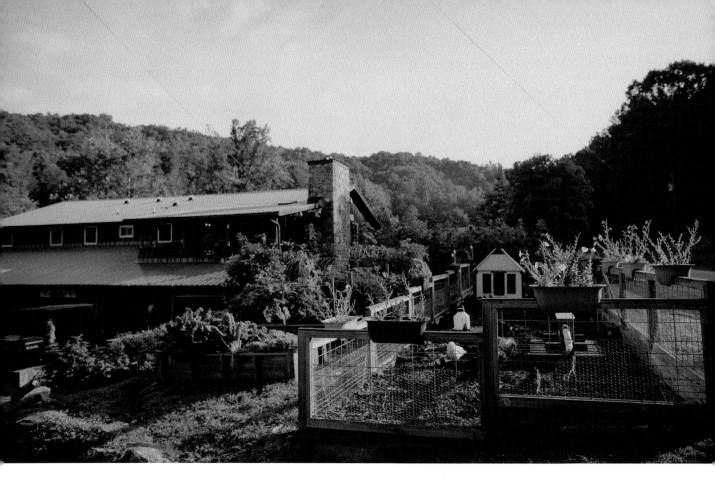

- *Color crops:* tomatoes, eggplant, peppers, radishes, carrots, cucumbers

There are lots of reasons to use a Container Garden besides having limited space—although that is the main reason. If you're living in a condo or an apartment, or if you don't have any usable land for growing, then a Container Garden is your only option.

But beyond that, Container Gardens are super easy to start and maintain, so they are a wonderful choice for starting small if you feel intimidated by the idea of growing your food. They are also portable, which means you can take your garden with you if you're renting or you might be moving in the near future.

How to Make It Happen

When you're ready to build your Container Garden, start by gathering the few supplies you'll need. Those will include:

- *Your containers.* See some of the options listed on page 45.
- *Organic potting soil.* We like a brand called Coco Loco by Bush Doctor.
- *Seeds or plant starts.* We recommend plant starts, which are just baby plants that have been growing for a few weeks. These are a little more expensive than seeds but are easier to grow. You can buy them at your local gardening shop or big-box hardware store. (If you can't

find starts or you prefer seeds, that's no problem—it will just take a little longer to harvest.)

- *Watering supplies.* Use a watering can for just a few containers or a wand or gardening hose if you've got lots of containers.

Step 1. Fill each container with potting soil to about 1.5 inches from the top.

Step 2. Locate the best spot for your Container Garden. You need to place your containers in a place that will get plenty of sun, which is typically the south side of your home, porch, or yard. (Or even the sills of your south-facing windows.)

Step 3. Plant your seeds or starts. For starts, just ease them gently into the soil until only the stem is poking out. For seeds, poke them right into the soil. Follow the spacing recommendations on your seed packet, but it won't hurt to plant multiple seeds as they might not all grow and you can weed out the weaker ones later.

Step 4. Water slightly. Consider using what's called a Fogg-It nozzle for seeds or very young sprouts as it won't wash away your seeds. Use just enough water to keep the soil moist. Continue to give at least 1 inch of water every week as the plant grows, maintaining an ever-so-slightly-moist soil throughout the growing period. That's really important because Container Gardens run the risk of drying out.

(See my Sticky Finger soil test on page 54 for another helpful tip.)

Step 5 (for seeds). Once your plants are about 1 inch tall, weed out the smaller shoots and keep only your best plants.

Step 6. At least once a week, pull out any weeds you see. You can do this by hand or with a small handheld hoe if you have a bigger Container Garden like my raised beds.

Step 7. It's harvesttime! If you're growing basil, spinach, salad greens, lettuces, kale, or other leafy plants, harvest the outer leaves as needed, but always leave at least three remaining. Other leaves will grow from the center of the plant, so you can have a perpetual harvest over several weeks.

Step 8. Once the plant stops growing and starts to wilt, that means it's finished growing. Harvest the remaining produce, throw out the unused plant, and start over if you're still in the growing season. (Reminder: you can check the growing seasons for your climate with a quick search online.) Or allow the soil to rest until the next growing season. If possible, move the containers to a sheltered area during the off-season.

That's it! Gardening can be that small (and easy). Growing your own food doesn't have to be this grandiose thing, and you don't need a 5-acre spread. Just a simple pot with a plant will do for getting you well on your way toward your food-growing dreams.

Raised Beds

I mentioned earlier that Rebekah and I have several raised beds as part of the gardens on our homestead. These are large wooden boxes that we've set on the ground and filled with logs (or wood chips), soil, and compost—which means they're basically Container Gardens on steroids.

I started using raised beds several years ago when our community got twice its normal amount of rain during the spring, which ended up washing out Rebekah's beloved tomatoes. Since then, I've come to love them as a gardening system because they bring a lot of benefits to the table and are virtually indestructible.

For one thing, raised beds are a beautiful addition to any home or garden. Combining the organic growth of whatever you choose to plant with the sharp cuts and grains of the wooden beds brings a unique look. For another thing, raised beds get your garden up off the ground, which adds protection not only from flooding or soggy soil, but also from animals or people stomping all over what you're trying to grow. Also, raised beds require very little work once you get them built, filled, and planted—I'm talking less than ten minutes of maintenance a week.

Finally, raised beds can produce a huge amount of food in even a small space. This is especially true if you plant in layers—for example, by having leafy greens at the bottom of the bed, tomatoes growing over the top, and containers attached to the sides for extra growing space. Whatever you can grow in a Container Garden, you can grow it at a much

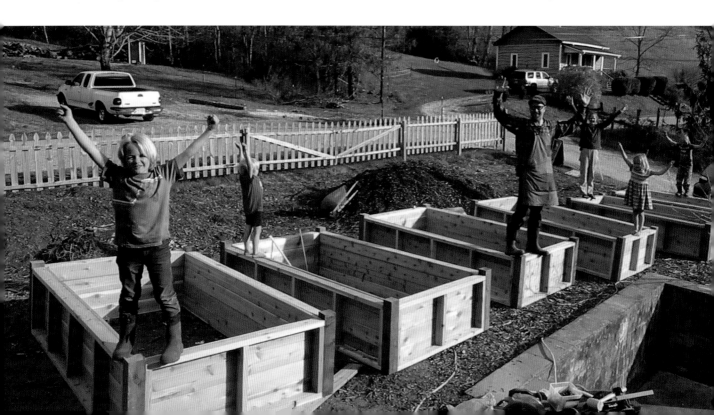

larger scale in raised beds. Also, you can use raised beds to grow pretty much anything that fits in a Bulletproof Garden (see below) or Crop Garden (see page 56).

If you want to learn more about raised beds, and even get step-by-step instructions for building them (supply list and all), check out TheRootedLife.com/Resources.

The Bulletproof Garden

One of my favorite experiences on our homestead is watching the children run around the grounds and interact with our gardens. I love the way they squat down on their heels and instinctively reach out to feel the different textures of leaves, stems, flowers, dirt, and fruits. I smile when they poke their heads down there for a better view—or when they look up at me, eyes wide, and tell me about some new bud or bug.

So, as lovely and efficient as raised beds can be, I'll always have a soft spot in my heart for gardens that are directly connected to the ground.

If you've got even a little space on your property or yard and you're ready to start growing in the ground, the Bulletproof Garden is a great way to start. I call it "bulletproof" because this system is quick, easy, inexpensive, and works just about anywhere.

Oh, and of course it grows a whole bunch of healthy, nutritious food!

The Bulletproof Garden is different from a Container Garden or raised beds in that it's

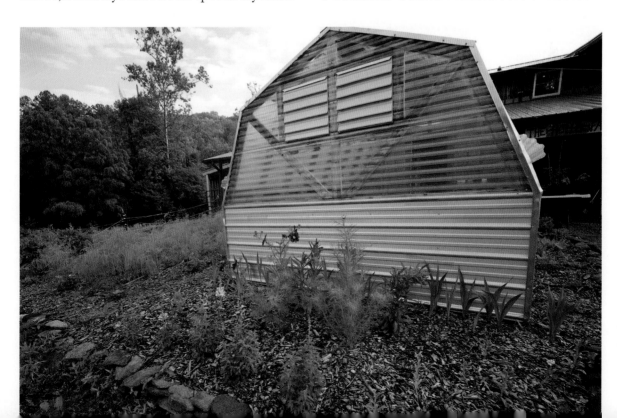

planted directly in the ground. However, that doesn't mean you have to get out your shovel or spade. In fact, leave those in the shed! One of the common mistakes people make when they start growing their own food is thinking they should till or plow or in some way chop up the ground before they plant. In reality, tilling wreaks havoc on the biological life in your soil, which in turn causes problems for your plants. Don't do it!

Instead, you'll build a Bulletproof Garden by adding mulch and compost *on top* of your soil and then planting underneath that mixture. That way your soil keeps its integrity and maintains a healthy biome, and the roots of your plants have a nice, firm foundation in which to take hold. Best of all, no digging for you!

There's more good news. Because the Bulletproof Garden is heavily mulched, you won't have to do nearly as much watering as in a typical garden. You'll also have a lot fewer weeds, and your plants will be stronger and grow longer.

Speaking of growing, here's what you can plant and harvest in a Bulletproof Garden:

- *Herbs:* oregano, dill, spearmint, peppermint, parsley, chives, cilantro, basil, thyme, sage, fennel, chamomile, lavender, rosemary, wheatgrass
- *Vegetables:* lettuces, kale, Swiss chard, broccoli, cabbages, tomatoes, eggplant, peppers, radishes, carrots, cucumbers, corn
- *Squashes:* spaghetti squash, acorn squash, pumpkin, yellow squash, zucchini
- *Melons:* cantaloupes, watermelons

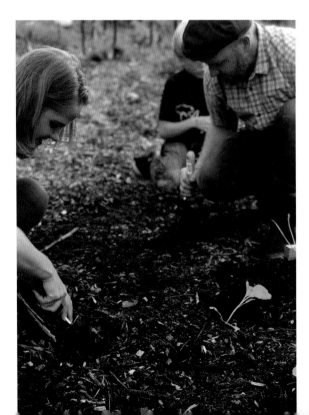
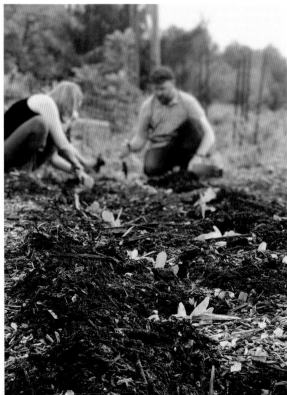

Ready to plant? First, you'll need to gather a few supplies.

What You'll Need

In terms of location, you'll need a mostly flat patch of ground for your Bulletproof Garden; I recommend somewhere in the ballpark of 4 by 8 feet. Pick a place that gets a lot of good sun. And remember, it's best to start as close to your front door as you can. That will prevent the garden from becoming "out of sight, out of mind," and it will be much more convenient for maintenance and harvesting.

When you've got the right spot, mow or trim the grass as low as you can—and keep the grass trimmings for mulch. Once again, don't dig up anything or till the ground. If you want to be exact, use some stakes and string to mark out exactly where the garden will be placed.

Keep in mind that you don't have to limit yourself to just one Bulletproof Garden bed. You can create and plant several beds at the same time and scale up your harvest with only a little bit of extra effort. If you have multiple gardens, make sure to leave 18 to 24 inches of pathways between beds so you can access everything.

Here are the other supplies you'll need to get started:

- *4 x 8 feet of nontoxic weed barrier.* WeedGuard Plus from Arbico Organics is a great option, and one package of 24 x 24 feet will be enough for several beds.

- *10 cubic feet of compost.* Compost is a natural soil amendment that will go a long way toward ensuring the successful growth of your plants. And 10 cubic feet will give you enough to spread 4 inches high over your entire bed.

- *10 cubic feet of grass clippings, organic straw, or leaves.* This will serve as a mulch around your plants to retain moisture, suppress weeds, and eventually add organic matter to your soil as they break down. I prefer grass clippings because they can be easily accessed from your yard and are easy to work with. (You can also use wood shavings or wood chips.) How much is 10 cubic feet of clippings? Well, enough to cover the garden with 4 inches of clippings.

- *Plant starts.* Instead of planting seeds directly in the ground, you're going to buy plant starts that are well on their way to success. Those who are more advanced gardeners can grow their own starts in a greenhouse before transplanting them into the garden. (Yes, I know starts are more expensive than seeds, but paying $6 for a tomato plant that will yield $60 worth of tomatoes is a great deal!) Trust me, this will make your life so much easier and will give you a much better chance at success.

- *Hand trowel.* This is for digging small holes to transplant your starts into the soil.
- *Up to 5 pounds of food scraps (optional).* This is worm food, which is important because worms do a good job of digging and aerating your soil and adding their manure (vermicompost), which is a wonderful thing for your garden.
- *Lead-free garden hose and nozzle.* You'll be watering your garden as you build and watering the plants as they grow. I love the quality of the Water Right hose, but any drinking-safe hose will work.

I do need to say one word here about spacing. Different plants take up different amounts of space in your garden, so you'll need to make a plan before purchasing your starts. Just to give an example, you can grow three or four lettuce plants in 1 square foot of soil, but only one cabbage plant in the same amount of space. Check the instructions on each plant start before you buy to get an idea of how much space will be required. Or, check out my handy Garden Spacing Guide at the back of this book (page 194).

One more thought: I strongly recommend you plan to grow about 25 percent more food than you need. That's because some plants may not thrive, some may get devoured by bugs, some may get prematurely plucked by precocious chiddlers, and so on. If you plan to grow more than you need, you won't feel as stressed when something goes wrong. And if you do end up with extra food at harvesttime? Your relatives and neighbors will likely be very happy to take it off your hands!

How to Make It Happen

Once you've mowed and staked the perfect spot—lots of sun but still as close to your front door as possible—you're ready to get planting. Here are the basic steps to follow for your brand-new Bulletproof Garden:

Step 1. If you're using food scraps, scatter them directly on the ground as food for the worms.

Step 2. Spread your compost evenly throughout the garden, aiming for a depth of about 4 inches. Yes, spread it right over any remaining grass or lawn. Give the compost a good watering—enough to soak it but not wash it away.

Step 3. Lay down your weed barrier, one or two sheets thick, to cover the entire garden, then soak the whole garden again. All this watering adds weight to the material so it won't blow away, and it also creates a nice moist environment for your thirsty plants.

Step 4. Place your 10 cubic feet of grass clippings (or other mulch) on top of the weed paper and wet everything again. Remember, that should spread out to about 4 inches deep.

Step 5. Now it's time to plant! First, dig a hole through the mulch, weed paper,

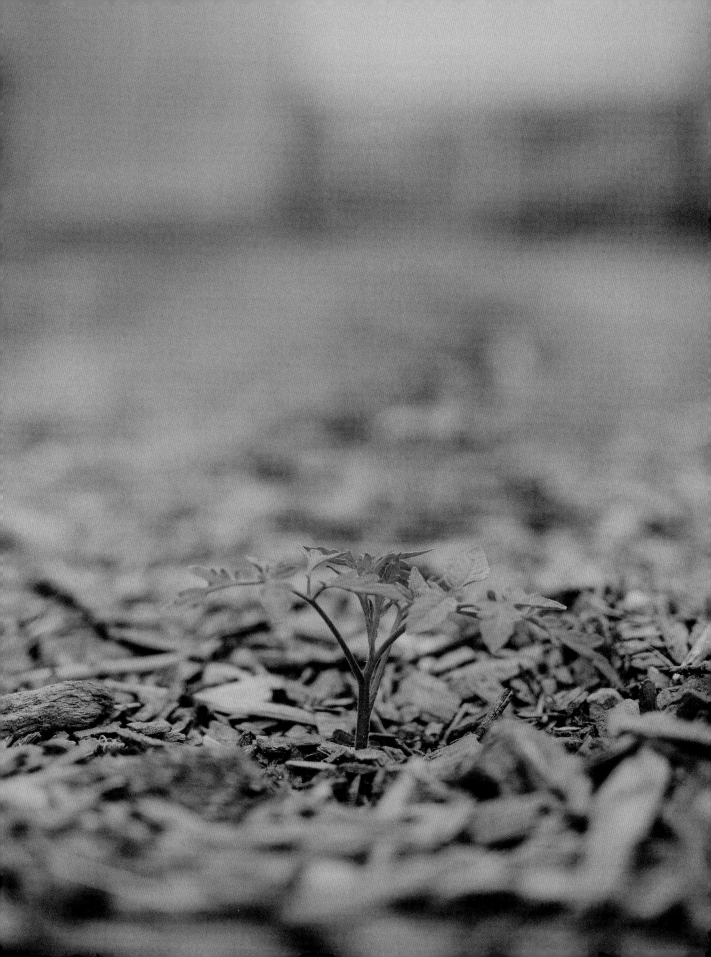

and compost for each plant—going deep enough into the soil to place your plant. Place the plant start directly in the hole so that just the stem is sticking up. Don't worry about packing or compressing the mulch around it. Keeping things a little loose is best.

Watering. When you first plant your starts, give them about an inch of water to help them cope with the transplant stress. After that, you'll need to monitor your moisture levels. In general, gardens need 1 inch of water per week, but a cool thing about the Bulletproof Garden is that all that mulch helps retain moisture.

If you watered your compost as instructed, you probably don't need to water right away, but if you forgot, then go ahead and give each plant an inch of "rain."

Here's a quick tip for figuring out the right amount to water: Find an empty tin can and mark out an inch, then "water" that can the way you would typically water your garden—use the same watering can, hose, or sprinkler, and time yourself doing it. When you figure out how long it takes to add an inch of water to the can, you'll know how long to water each section of your garden.

One more tip: I call this the Sticky Finger soil test. If you want to find out whether your soil is getting the right amount of water, stick your finger deep into the mulch, hold it for a couple of seconds, then pull it out. If your finger is dry, you're not watering enough. If your finger is wet—like, muddy and soaked—you're watering too much. If your finger has wet soil sticking to it, everything is just right.

You can go weeks without watering if it's raining where you are. Even then, the Sticky Finger soil test will give you a good indication of how your soil is doing.

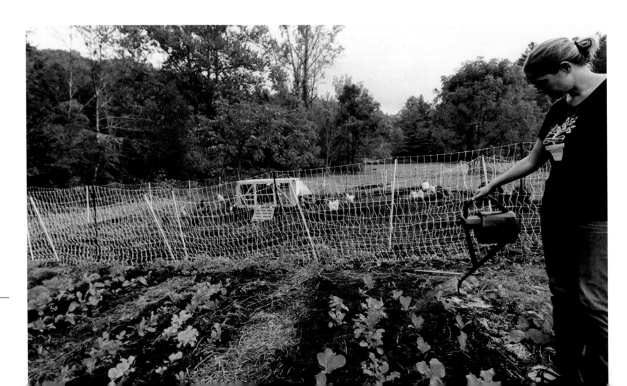

Weeding. One of the great benefits of the Bulletproof Garden is that your weed barrier and mulch will effectively smother most of the weeds that try to grow. Still, it's good to check things once a week and pull out anything that shouldn't be growing there. Again, because of the layers of compost and mulch, the weeds will pull out super easily. I love this garden!

Harvesting. This will be your biggest job with the Bulletproof Garden. Seriously! You'll be amazed at how much you can grow once everything gets going. Speaking of which, make sure to check on your plants regularly once the harvest starts so you can claim as much of the bounty as possible. (We'll talk more about harvesting and what to do after the harvest in Chapter 8.)

That's it! That's all you need to start growing an incredible amount of food every year with a lovely, easy, abundant Bulletproof Garden.

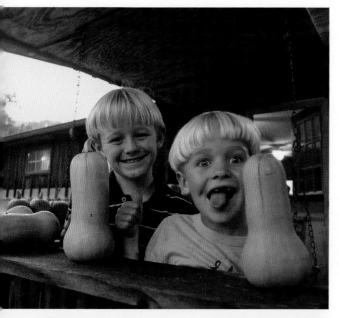

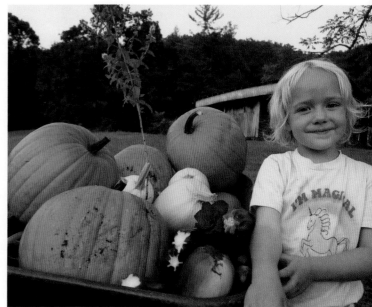

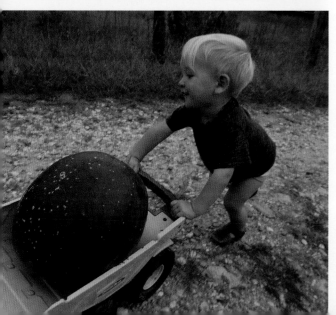

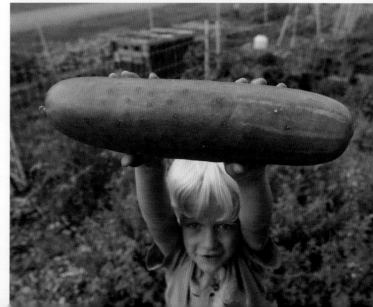

Crop Gardens

Rebekah and I have had several big, transitional moments on our journey toward the rooted life. Buying our first livestock was a good example. So was the first time we harvested eggs from our chickens (more on that in a later chapter). But in terms of the overall effect on our lives, our wallets, and cultivating our own health and wellness, I'm not sure anything has been a bigger transition than starting our Crop Gardens.

One of the reasons our Crop Gardens felt like such a big transition was the amount of work they required on the front end. As you'll see below, they're very different from Container Gardens or even the Bulletproof Garden. But the main reason our Crop Gardens felt so different was the sheer amount of food they produced—and keep producing!

I remember the first time I loaded up an entire wheelbarrow with a single crop from a single harvest. I loved that feeling! And when I did a little quick calculating and figured out how much it would cost to buy all that squash at the grocery store, I almost shouted for joy. It was that special.

What is a Crop Garden? At the core, it's a scaled-up version of the Bulletproof Garden, although there are some key differences. For one thing, you will need to break up the ground and shape your garden beds the first time you plant a Crop Garden. (But only the first time!) You'll also need to use seeds and create your own plant starts in order to keep costs down. And you'll need a plan for harvesting, storing, and preserving all the bounty you'll grow.

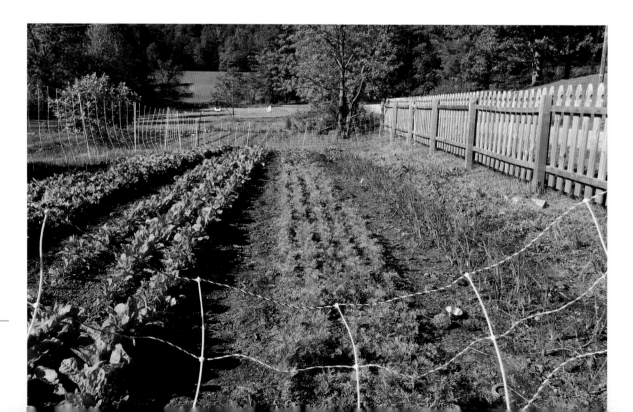

You should consider a Crop Garden if:

- You want to grow the majority of your own food—I'm talking at least 75 percent of your produce during the growing season.
- You're ready for the most efficient style of gardening (the same kind used by the pros).
- You have a relatively flat area of land that gets good sun and is roughly 24 x 50 feet.
- You are willing and able to handle a higher degree of manual labor—building beds, spreading compost, weeding, loading up harvests, and so on.

If all that sounds good to you, let's plant!

What You'll Need

The biggest thing you'll need for a Crop Garden is the land itself. The instructions and measurements I've included here will require a 24 x 50-foot space. That will produce seven beds that are 30 inches wide and 50 feet long, with 12 inches of space between beds.

Why 50 feet? It's not a magic number, but a lot of the gardening supplies you'll buy come in lengths of a hundred feet. So, it's easy to cut those in half. Also, I like my beds to be 30 inches wide because it's easy to straddle that much space and reach from side to side when you're planting, weeding, checking, or

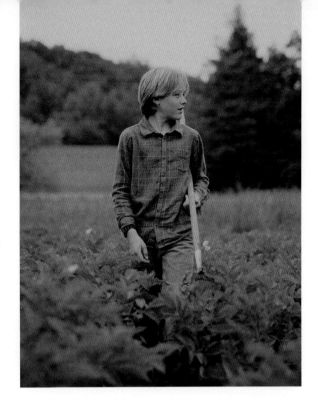

harvesting. And many gardening tools are set up for a standard 30-inch garden.

Keep in mind that each of those seven beds can hold multiple rows of crops, depending on how much spacing those crops need. For example, one bed that is 30 inches wide and 50 feet long can hold five rows of carrots. Each crop has different spacing requirements, so you'll need to keep track of the instructions on the seed packets. (Or check the Garden Spacing Guide on page 194.)

Here are the supplies you'll need to find ahead of time for a successful Crop Garden:

- *Walking tractor or tiller.* You'll only need this machine once in order to break ground and begin your first garden. Chances are you can borrow one or rent one since you'll really only need it once.

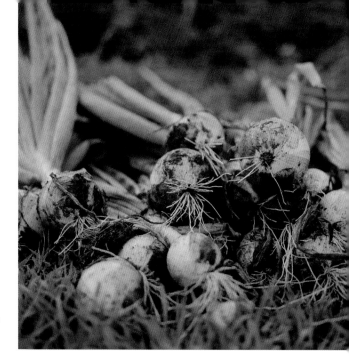

Or, if you know of a local gardener who already has this equipment, you can hire him or her to do the work for you.

- *Compost, plus a wheelbarrow and a shovel.* You'll need 7 cubic yards to spread over all seven beds (1 cubic yard of compost per bed). You can fit 2 cubic yards of compost in a regular pickup truck bed, or closer to 4 cubic yards if you have a truck and trailer. But I'd advise you to go online to find a local source that delivers, such as a landscape supply store.

- *A hard rake, soft rake, and flat shovel.* These tools help shape the beds and pull out weeds or other unneeded plant material.

- *A hoe.* We prefer what's called a stirrup hoe. With a stirrup hoe you can clip the weeds going forward and backward. We like the 5-inch stirrup hoe from Johnny's Selected Seeds because its small blade size lets us easily hoe between most plants.

- *A broadfork.* This is for aerating and hydrating the soil. I like the 12-inch People's broadfork from Meadow Creature.

- *Silage tarps.* These tarps are UV-resistant plastic sheets for covering bare soil to prepare it for planting. These can be ordered online from Johnny's Selected Seeds or Farmers Friend in a 24 x 100-foot size. (Cut it in half to make two tarps.)

- *Stakes and twine.* You'll use stakes and twine to shape and plant your beds in straight lines.

- *A gridder.* If you have the resources, you can use a gridder from Neversink Farm to mark off where you'll plant each start. Otherwise, space out the plants by setting up a straight line with twine and measuring down the twine as you plant.

- *Seeds and other supplies to make your own plant starts.* Because you're going to be growing hundreds of plants, it would get very expensive to buy plant starts. Instead, buy seeds and use a greenhouse or other method to grow your own plant starts (described in the next section), which can then be transplanted into the Crop Garden beds.

Growing Your Own Starts

If creating your own plant starts sounds complicated, don't worry about it. You can absolutely make it happen, and you'll save yourself a bundle of money in the process.

First, you will need a few supplies:

- *Soil.* We use a local mix from our gardening supply store but have also used the nationally distributed Coco Loco brand with great success. One bag of soil (2 cubic feet) will give you about ten soil trays, which is 360 plant starts.
- *Soil blocker.* This is a device that turns loose soil into compact, movable blocks. We use a 2-inch blocker for all of our starts. We got ours online from Johnny's Selected Seeds.
- *Soil block trays.* These are for efficiently holding, stacking, and moving your soil blocks (and eventually your plant starts, once the seeds are planted). You can buy these premade, or you can find plans for our soil trays at TheRootedLife.com/ Resources. (Each of our trays holds thirty-six soil blocks.)
- *Mixing tub.* You can use a wheelbarrow to mix your soil and make your blocks, or you can buy something premade. We have a 25-gallon Tuff Stuff tub.
- *Greenhouse.* It's very helpful to have a greenhouse to keep your starts safe from the big, bad world while they are still young. Again, there are many premade

greenhouses that are surprisingly affordable. Ours is from Ana White. Or, you can find plans to build my Slapped-Together Greenhouse at TheRootedLife.com/Resources.

- *Mist waterer.* You need to be careful not to water with a strong hose at first, or you risk washing out the seeds. Use a mist waterer to keep everything safe. We have a Dramm waterer.
- *Outdoor table.* This is for "hardening" your plant starts when it gets close to the time for transplanting them into your garden. Any wood, plastic, or metal table should do. Just make sure it's solid and can hold some weight. We have a few plastic folding tables from Sam's Club.

When you're ready to start your starts, dump a quarter or half of your soil into the mixing tub. Mix the soil around while adding water until you have a brownie-mix consistency.

Next, fill your soil blocker by pressing the blocker into the tub of soil. It's good to push down into at least 3 or 4 inches of soil. That way any extra soil will clear out and you'll be able to really compress the soil into your blocks. If your blocks are crumbly and won't stick together, you need to add more water. If your soil won't stay in the blocker or hold form, you have too much water. In that case just add a bit more soil.

Fill your soil block trays with soil blocks. Then drop your seeds on top of each soil block. Rebekah and I don't cover the seeds since we like them to get plenty of air. Others cover the seeds slightly with soil. Both methods seem to work fine.

About a week before you plan to transplant the starts into the garden, begin "hardening" them off by placing them on your outside table during the day. This will literally harden the soil blocks so they will stay together better when planted. (Bring the starts back inside for the night during this week.)

How to Make It Happen

Whenever you're planting a garden, it's important to make a plan and be intentional about what you want to grow—but this is especially critical with a Crop Garden. Remember, start from the door of your heart and plant what you are most likely to eat.

Planning a Crop Garden also means you need to be aware of seasons and timing. You don't want to plant anything until after the last possible frost date for your climate zone, unless you plan on covering your crops to protect them from frost (see Chapter 4 for more information). A major advantage of Crop Gardens is that you can plant multiple crops throughout the year—you can plant a spring garden and harvest the produce, then plant a summer garden and harvest again, all before the growing season ends. For that reason, you need to plant early enough to do your final harvest before things start to freeze.

Be sure to take advantage of the flattest, sunniest spot for your Crop Garden. Being close to the house isn't as important in this system as you typically won't visit it as much as your other gardens. Plus, you'll usually have more work (and harvest) with every visit, which makes a longer commute to work worth the effort.

Finally, it's important to be aware of spacing when you plan out your Crop Garden. You need to know how many plants you will sow in each row, which means you need to understand how much room each of those plants requires. Again, check out my Garden Spacing Guide on page 194.

To give you an example of what all this looks like, here's what Rebekah and I might plant in a typical spring garden:

- ½ bed of collards (150 starts)
- ½ bed of Swiss chard (150 starts)
- 1 bed of lettuces (288 starts) with a couple of feet of spinach (24 starts)
- 2 beds of cabbages (200 starts)
- 1 bed of carrots (hundreds, if not thousands of seeds)
- ½ bed of beets (150 starts)
- ½ bed of turnips (150 starts)
- 1 bed of broccoli (44 starts) with 6 feet of Brussels sprouts (6 starts)

See what I mean about the magnitude of Crop Gardens? That's a lot of food! But that's only the first planting. After we harvest all that goodness, we can replant the same Crop Garden for the summer, like this:

- 1 bed of tomatoes (50 starts)
- ½ bed of peppers (50 starts)
- ½ bed of herbs
- 1 bed of cucumbers (50 starts)
- 2 beds of green beans (400 direct seeded)
- 2 beds of watermelons (50 starts)

Boom! Are you starting to see how Crop Gardens can provide the majority of your family's food over a given year? And that doesn't even include what you can grow in a Winter Harvest Garden (see Chapter 4).

Okay, enough showing off. Here are the steps you need to take to get started for yourself.

Step 1. Order your seeds anytime during the winter. You'll want to begin turning those seeds into plant starts about four weeks prior to transplanting them into your Crop Garden. You can find more details on how to grow your own seed starts at TheRootedLife.com/Resources.

Step 2. If you have silage tarps available during the winter, put them down on your Crop Garden area for two or three months to kill the grass and other vegetation. If you get your silage tarps in the spring, you'll likely need to keep them on the ground for a month or two. (You can also mow down any grass as low as possible before you add the tarps.) These tarps will block the sun

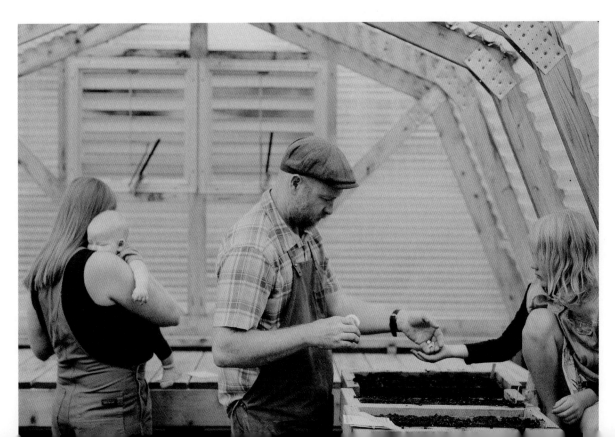

from getting to the grass, weeds, and any other existing vegetation, so it will all die out and start to decompose—which is great for the soil.

Step 3. This is optional, but you may want to get your soil tested to see if it needs any supplements or amendments. Our soil is acidic clay, for example, so we add a 40-pound bag of lime and a 40-pound bag of gypsum every year to address that issue and keep it healthy. If you do a test and need to add supplements, put them in before you cover the beds with your silage tarp.

Step 4. At least two weeks before planting, you need to shape your beds. Start by removing your silage tarp. Rent or borrow a walking tractor with a rotary plow option. This is the best way to break in new ground with minimum impact on the soil life. It turns the soil more than mixing it. Afterward, the ground will now be workable with hand tools for shaping the beds. A rototiller will do if you can't get ahold of the walking tractor with rotary plow; it will just be a bit more damaging to your soil. Certainly not the end of the world, though.

Mark your beds with twine and use a flat shovel to dig out your paths, spreading that soil where your 30-inch beds will be. Digging out each path and tossing the dirt on your bed does the actual shaping of the garden bed.

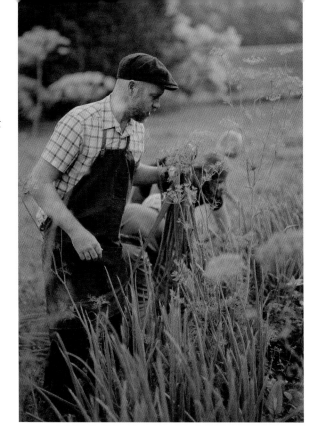

Step 5. Now add about 1 cubic yard of compost per bed. That's about five wheelbarrow loads per bed. We drop a wheelbarrow load every 10 feet, then spread the piles evenly over the bed with shovels and hard rakes.

Now cover again with the silage tarp until you're ready for planting. The soil disturbance will probably bring up a good amount of weed seeds, which will sprout now that they have access to air and light. So it's a great idea to cover your newly shaped garden beds for at least two weeks to prevent those weeds from growing.

Step 6. Rake out any weeds, grass, or other remaining vegetation. Then use your broadfork on your beds to aerate and hydrate the soil. This gives you the benefits of tilling the ground without damaging the biome of your soil. (If you don't know how to broadfork, you can find my preferred methods at TheRootedLife.com/Resources.)

Step 7. Use twine to lay out your straight lines for planting. (Or, if possible, use the Neversink gridder.)

Step 8. It's time to plant! Just as in the Bulletproof Garden, use a hand trowel to dig a small hole for each of your plant starts. Then set the start in the ground so that the soil is level with the stem.

Step 9. Give your plant starts a generous watering (an inch or more) in the days before and after you transplant. That will help them get over the stress of being moved.

Weeding. Use your hoe once a week to keep the weeds at bay. If you've really got a lot of weed growth that first year, you may need to rake twice a week.

Watering. In general, give your crops about an inch of water every week to keep them strong and healthy (skipping weeks when it rains). Unlike the Bulletproof Garden, however, watering a Crop Garden requires more than a single can or hose. You'll need a system to water your different rows and beds without too much trouble, and below I describe several options to choose from.

Also, remember the Sticky Finger soil test (see page 54)! That's a great way to quickly determine whether your crops are getting the right amount of water throughout the growing season.

Harvesting. We'll talk a lot more about harvesting in the next chapter, plus what you'll need to do to maintain your gardens after the growing season is over. For now, just remember that harvesting a Crop Garden will mean a lot of work and a whole lot of food!

Watering Your Crop Gardens

Crop Gardens are large enough that you don't want to try watering them by hand. Trust me. Instead, I strongly recommend you purchase or set up a system that will allow you to water the crops evenly without taking up a whole lot of your time.

To make that happen, you'll need a few supplies:

- *A high-quality garden hose.* I like the Water Right brand. Make sure you get a hose that's long enough to stretch from your spigot and still reach all areas of the garden.
- *An automated sprinkler.* An Orbit garden sprinkler can be picked up at big-box hardware stores and is able to water an entire 24 x 50-foot garden plot from one side. If you need something bigger and more heavy-duty, the Raintower Sprinkler from Irrigation King will cover one garden plot extremely well— but can also water two garden plots from the side of one of the plots.

Remember my tin can trick: mark an inch inside an empty can, and then "water" the can until you accumulate an inch of water. That's how long you need to water your Crop Gardens each week (assuming it doesn't rain). Because Crop Gardens are so large, you may need to experiment with positioning your watering system so that you cover the whole garden.

Here are a few more rules of thumb for effective watering:

- When possible, do your watering in the morning before the sun gets intense. This means less evaporation, and it also gives time for the water to soak into the soil before nightfall—which helps prevent fungus.
- Watering deeply is more important than watering frequently. Longer, deeper watering encourages deep root growth as opposed to shallow root growth from light waterings. This goes a long way toward growing strong, healthy plants.
- Skip watering when the temperature is below 40°F.
- Remember the Sticky Finger soil test (page 54) if you aren't certain whether your soil is sufficiently watered.

Dealing with Bugs and Pests

Rebekah and I don't use any type of pesticides or chemicals on or around our gardens. One of the main reasons we grow our own food is to avoid that kind of pollution and all the health problems it can cause—for us, our animals, and our planet.

Still, we can't wish away the bugs, and people often ask me how to deal with pests in a natural, healthy way. So, let me go through some important thoughts on what I know is an important issue to many people.

Grow more than you need. The biggest thing you can do to handle bugs and pests is to grow more than you need and be willing to share. Yes, even share with the bugs! They're going to get some, and you'll have a lot less stress if you just open your mind to that reality from the beginning. Whenever I see bugs getting into one of my plants, I think of that as my Organic Stamp of Approval. If my food is clean enough for the bugs to want it, that means it's clean enough for me and my family.

I typically recommend planting 25 percent more than you need. That's the easiest way to deal with bugs and other wildlife. Thankfully, if your soil is healthy and you take other precautions (see below), bugs will have a limited effect on your overall food production.

Grow in good soil. The good news is you don't have to wave the white flag and let bugs eat all your crops. Bugs are a big problem for industrial farms because the soil they use has become so stripped and unhealthy over the years that the plants themselves are unhealthy—which means they are prone to being overwhelmed by bugs. Entire crops can be lost when unhealthy plants are unable to defend themselves.

When you plant your garden, however, you're going to be using good soil that is composted and well mulched. Your soil will have a healthy biome and microorganisms because it has not been stripped by years of overuse. That good soil will produce strong, healthy plants that are capable of defending themselves against bugs and other pests. Watering regularly will also go a long way toward keeping your plants strong enough and healthy enough to protect themselves against bugs.

Use nets if necessary. Brassica vegetables—cabbages, broccoli, cauliflower, Brussels sprouts, kale, bok choy, and so on—are especially prone to attacks from bugs. If you are growing a lot of those plants, you may want to invest in some bug nets. You can simply lay the bug nets over the top of your crops and use some weights to hold them down. Or, you can build a little arch with wires and drape the net over a whole garden area.

If possible, keep some areas of your property wild. If you have untamed land on your property, or if you've got woods around your gardens, that can be a great tool for dealing with pests. That's because it allows space for other animals who are predators of those pests to thrive. Birds, bats, spiders, and larger bugs such as praying mantises will all help you control bugs on your property if they have a place to live. I know bugs can be intimidating and even scary. Take wasps, for example. We don't kill them if they get in our house.

Instead, I carefully catch them in a jar and release them outside. Why? Because wasps eat aphids, which wreak havoc on all kinds of garden goodness.

Harvest your bugs. This is a classic example of turning a problem into a solution. If you have a lot of bugs munching on your plants—maybe some squash bugs, for example—go out to your garden in the morning with a bucket of water. Harvest those bugs by picking them off the plants and tossing them in the water, which means they can't fly away. Then, when you've got all the bugs you can see, toss that water over to your chickens to feed on. That way you're turning those bugs into healthy chicken and eggs! (If you don't have chickens, just let the bugs drown and then dump the water.)

———————

There you have my three systems for growing your own food: Container Gardens, Bulletproof Gardens, and Crop Gardens. No matter where you are on your journey toward the rooted life, one of these options—or a combination of two or even all three—is guaranteed to help you cultivate health and wellness like you've never experienced.

Gardening Basics

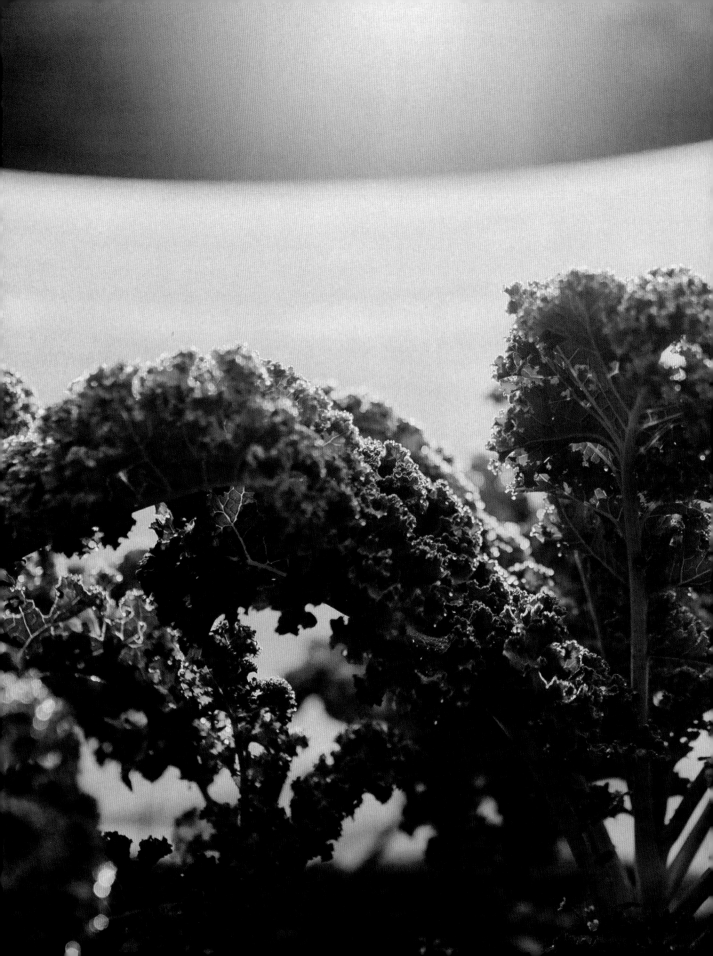

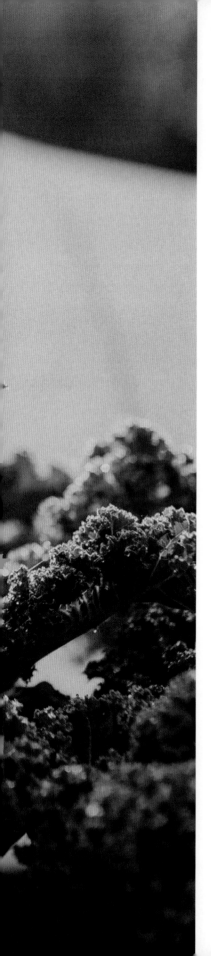

CHAPTER 4

The Winter Harvest Garden

When Rebekah and I first started embracing the rooted life and building up the different elements of our homestead, we read a lot of books. We still read quite a bit, of course, but in those early years we were especially hungry for knowledge. Thankfully, Rebekah has quite a knack for finding just the right book at just the right moment when we are working to solve a problem or about to try something new.

One of the most influential books we discovered was *The New Organic Grower* by Eliot Coleman. Man, I dug through his work from cover to cover, over and over again. His insights and practical instructions played a huge role in the methods we adopted for growing our own food.

I remember one day in particular when I came across Eliot's thoughts about harvesting food in the winter. My ears perked up. After all, this guy was growing his crops *in Maine*!

At first I thought he must have invested a ton of money in building a gigantic greenhouse with a bunch of artificial lights and fancy heating systems. Nope. Eliot Coleman successfully gardens in the winter without supplemental heat or artificial lights. In fact, he's so successful he even flipped his garden routine one year to provide veggies to sell at the market in the winter while taking a break in the summer!

Wait a minute, Eliot! You're telling me I could have fresh veggies at Christmas dinner and beyond? No preservation?

As you can imagine, we were all over this idea. We started planning our Winter Harvest Garden right away, and we were able to start planting that summer. Wouldn't you know it? That Christmas we had an entire dinner direct from our homestead—roasted chicken, potatoes, and even *fresh* greens harvested on Christmas Eve.

We've continued to plant a Winter Harvest Garden almost every year, and we still love the feeling of having fresh food available at every season. There have been many times when I've put on my boots and trudged out through the snow to harvest some lettuce or cabbage for a fresh salad. I love that feeling!

Ready to learn how to do it?

Before You Start

Before you get planting, let's make sure we're on the same page regarding what a Winter Harvest Garden is and how it benefits you.

The basic idea here is to plant a garden late in the growing season so that you can harvest the produce all winter long. But you still need to plant early enough for those crops to get to a mature size before the days get colder and shorter, and growth slows dramatically. For that reason, determining the best time to plant your Winter Harvest Garden takes a little calculating.

The first thing to figure out is when your location gets down to ten hours of sunshine in a day. That's because plants need ten-plus hours of sunshine each day in order to grow. The more sunlight, the more growth—which is why farmers in Alaska can grow 81-pound cabbages, because the sun shines twenty hours a day in the summer. You can find out when your daylight gets down to ten hours a day by checking Solartopo.com, among other online resources.

Once you have that date, the next step is to determine what you want to plant. Unfortunately, this concept doesn't work with every type of crop. There are no tomatoes, cucumbers, or other heat-loving crops in our Winter Harvest Garden. Instead, you need to choose plants that do well in cold weather. Here are some of the most popular options: spinach, kale, cabbages, arugula, lettuces, Brussels sprouts, broccoli, turnips, carrots, radishes, collards, Swiss chard, parsley, sorrel, and beets.

When you know what you want to grow, determine how long it will take each type of plant to reach maturity. You can do that by checking the instructions on your seed packets or starts—then adding fifteen to twenty days. That's really important because plants don't grow as quickly in the fall as they do in the spring or summer. So, let's say you want to plant lettuce, which usually takes sixty days to mature. To harvest that lettuce in winter, you'll need to plan for seventy-five or eighty days before your ten hours of daylight date.

Here's a quick timeline of how this works in our Winter Harvest Garden, just to give you an example:

- Our time for ten hours of sunlight each day usually comes around Thanksgiving—the end of November.
- To plant quick-maturing crops such as lettuce, which normally takes sixty days to mature, we plan for eighty days in the winter. That means the latest we could plant those crops is early September— eighty days before Thanksgiving.
- To plant seeds and other longer-developing crops that would normally require 90 days to maturity, we plan for 110 days. That means the earliest we can start planting those crops is early August—110 days before Thanksgiving.
- Thus, our planting window is between early August and late September. By planting our crops within that window, we'll be golden for a winter harvest.

By now, you're probably looking for the catch. I mean, how can it be possible to grow fresh veggies when there's snow on the ground? Well, there is a catch. Kind of. It's not really a big deal. You can grow a Winter Harvest Garden from Georgia to Maine as long as you plant in the right window—but you will need to protect what you grow from frost and snow. And that typically means using simple covers such as tunnels (see the instructions below).

Now here's the best part: it's called a Winter Harvest Garden because that's all you have to do—harvest. There's no weeding. There's little or no watering once the weather turns cold. And winter means no bugs to deal with. In other words, other than your tunnels, this garden has practically no maintenance!

Sure, you'll probably need to cover your rows from time to time, depending on where you live. But that's not a big deal. And the reward for your (minimum) effort is harvesting fresh, healthy veggies all winter long.

I know you're excited about this potential bounty for your family, so let's plant!

What You'll Need

The plans and supply lists below are based on using the same beds as the Crop Gardens we covered in Chapter 3. So, we're talking about garden beds that are 30 inches wide and 50 feet long, with at least 12 inches of footpath between rows.

If you don't have that much land available to plant a Winter Harvest Garden, you can still grow your winter crops in raised beds, a Bulletproof Garden, or even Container

Gardens. You'll just need to find some additional (and maybe creative) ways to cover those gardens to protect your plants from frost and snow.

Just as with Crop Gardens, it's not cost-effective to buy hundreds of plant starts for a Winter Harvest Garden. (Also, plant starts can be tough to find in the fall.) Instead, you'll want to buy seeds and grow them into starts over a period of a few weeks.

Once your plant starts are ready, you'll transplant them into the beds of your Winter Harvest Garden in the same way as for a Crop Garden.

Next, as I mentioned earlier, you will need to cover your winter plants to protect them against frost and snow. So, let's quickly run through three options you can use to make that happen.

Mulch

There are several winter crops that grow below the ground, which means you don't have to use tunnels or other methods to protect them. Instead, you can just cover the beds with unsprayed hay or organic straw, and then let those crops grow. (Just make sure you apply that covering before the first frost in your area.)

Plants that can be covered this way include beets, carrots, and turnips.

Low Tunnels

This is the quickest—not to mention the most affordable and effective—way to cover and protect your aboveground crops during the winter months. Rebekah and I have used low tunnels for years now, ever since I first read Eliot Coleman's book, and we've had great success. It's amazing how easily you can get up and running with this system.

What is a low tunnel? It's a long, arched covering that extends the entire length of your garden beds. You'll set up the frame of each tunnel using ½-inch metal conduits stuck into the ground at each side of your beds, then you'll stretch a piece of Agribon covering over the frame. When there is snow in the forecast, you'll add greenhouse plastic to the frame as well.

Here are the supplies you'll need for one low tunnel, which will cover two garden beds that are 30 inches wide and 50 feet long, with a 12-inch footpath in the middle. If you want to cover more than two beds, you'll need to scale the supplies. (For example, if you want to cover four beds, just double the supply list below.)

- *Fifteen metal conduits that are each 10 feet long and ½ inch in diameter.* These make the frame for your tunnels. You'll use one conduit for each end of the tunnel, and then space out the rest about every 4 feet.
- *Pole bender.* You'll need this tool from Johnny's Selected Seeds to shape your metal conduits into arches.
- *A 10-foot-wide Agribon low cover for frost protection.* These might be available from

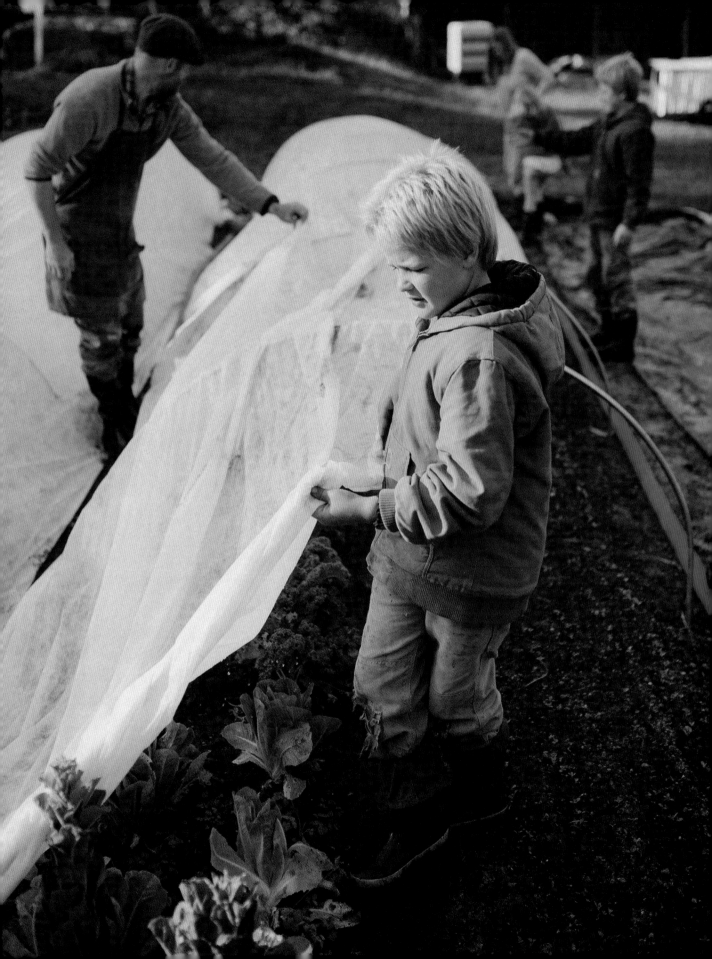

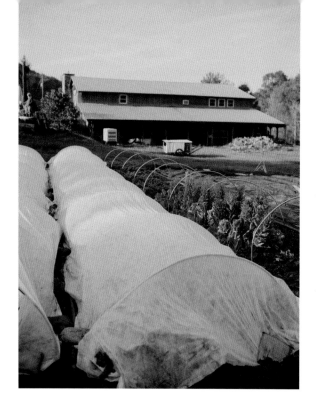

your local gardening store or landscape supply. We get ours online from Johnny's Selected Seeds.

- *A 10-foot-wide sheet of greenhouse plastic for snow protection.* Buy this from the same place as your Agribon. When you expect snow, simply add the sheeting over your tunnel frame for extra protection.
- *Fifty sandbags or other weights.* We use 10- to 14-inch sandbags (15-pound capacity) to hold the metal conduits in place and weigh down the coverings. You'll want a weight placed at each end of the tunnel and then the rest spaced out every 2 feet. We get the UV-resistant kind from Uline.com.
- *Sand for your sandbags.* You can buy sand in 50-pound bags from a hardware

store, or set up a delivery from a local landscape supply store.

I'll use low tunnels in my instructions below, because they really are the simplest way to protect your winter crops. Yes, there is some effort involved. But I can tell you from experience they still beat the pants off of running out to the grocery store for veggies every week during the winter months! Especially when you have severe weather.

However, if the Winter Harvest Garden is a concept you really enjoy, and you plan on doing this year after year, you might want to invest in high tunnels (see below). Yes, these are more expensive than low tunnels, but the ease of getting in and out will make them worth it in the long run.

High Tunnels

One of the disadvantages of low tunnels is that you can't walk through them. When you need to access your plants, or when you need to ventilate them (more on that below), you have to remove the weights from one side and pull back the covering. That's not a big deal, but it can be a minor annoyance if you get a lot of snow or if your weather fluctuates quite a bit.

So, one alternative is to build high tunnels, which are essentially long greenhouses that extend the entire length of your garden beds. Yes, I know I said at the beginning of this chapter that harvesting veggies in the winter doesn't require greenhouses—but that doesn't mean you *can't* use greenhouses! Besides, high tunnels are different from traditional greenhouses in that you don't have to heat them.

The big advantage for high tunnels is that they are stable—you don't have to take them down or add coverings when there's snow in the forecast. Another big advantage is that you can walk into these tunnels and easily access your crops.

The big disadvantage to high tunnels is the cost. They can be expensive, especially for large garden beds. But again, if this is something you plan to do long-term, the increase in production thanks to ease and accessibility will be well worth the expense. We're happy with our high tunnels from Growers Solution.

How to Make It Happen

Now that you've figured out which winter crops you want to grow, it's time to determine how much of each one you're going to plant. That will make a big difference in how many rows you plant, how to space out those rows, and how many low tunnels you need.

Remember, the most important principle here is to start at the door of your heart. Only plant what you enjoy eating! *Do not* grow anything you don't like. You'll thank me later. You just won't want to go out there and cover or ventilate that Swiss chard if you can't stand the stuff. Don't feel bad if the only thing you like is cabbage—just plant cabbages. Who cares what all the cool people are doing on Instagram?

Seriously, promise me you'll plant only what you like to eat.

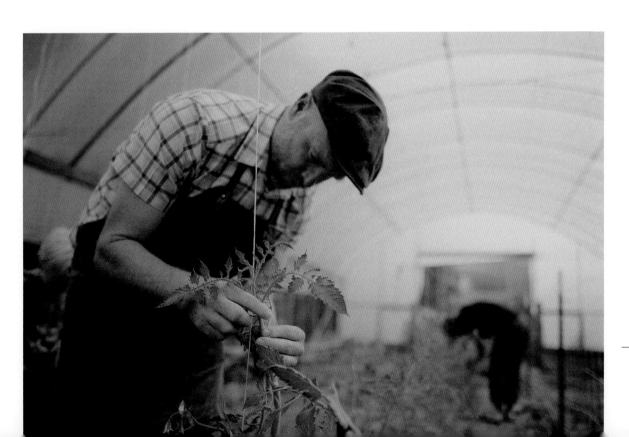

Also, remember to plant at least 25 percent more than you'll need. It might help to think about how much of a certain vegetable your family will eat over a four-month period, or roughly sixteen weeks. So, if you plant 150 kale plants, that will produce at least 150 kale bunches. You'll be harvesting all that over four months, which comes out to nine bunches of kale a week. For our family, that's plenty.

For the purposes of these instructions, I'll assume you're using an existing Crop Garden, which is what Rebekah and I do. That means you'll have seven garden rows available that are each 50 feet long and 30 inches wide. That's a lot of space to grow a lot of veggies!

For our family, we start our plans with kale, collards, Swiss chard, and lettuces. That's because those crops have pretty much the same spacing, which means they fit well together. We use three entire garden rows for those leafy greens, although sometimes we sneak something extra into part of those rows. (We might plant a few feet of spinach, for example, and cut back a little on lettuces.)

Next, we think through our wide-spaced crops: cabbages, broccoli, and Brussels sprouts. We love cabbages, and we can plant about a hundred of them in one garden row. Come harvesttime, that means four cabbages a week all through the winter—which again is plenty. We'll use another row for the broccoli and Brussels sprouts.

Finally, we save a couple of rows for crops that don't require tunnels. Since we really like carrots and they're so easy to cover (using organic straw or unsprayed hay), we give them an entire 50-foot row. Then we do another row with half beets and half turnips.

So, here's what our Winter Harvest Garden might look like:

- ½ bed of kale (150 starts)
- ½ bed of collards (150 starts)
- ½ bed of Swiss chard (150 starts)
- 1½ beds of lettuces (450 starts), with a couple of feet of spinach
- 1 bed of cabbages (100 starts)
- 1 bed of broccoli (44 starts), with 6 feet of Brussels sprouts (6 starts)
- 1 bed of carrots (hundreds, if not thousands of seeds)
- ½ bed of beets (150 starts)
- ½ bed of turnips (150 starts)

Yours will be different, of course, because you're going to plant what you like best! Also, if you are just getting started with harvesting in winter, I'd advise you to start with just two rows that require tunnels. That way you can get used to the process. (You can still add some rows with belowground crops that require only mulch for covering.)

Ready to plant? Here's a basic timeline you can follow. Remember, you'll determine your planting window based on when your home location starts to get less than ten hours of light a day. Details about each step can be found in Chapter 3.

Four weeks before planting. Start your seeds in soil blocks or something similar. If possible, start them in a vented greenhouse that includes a shade cloth. Remember, you're planting cold-hardy crops in the middle of the summer, so you'll need something to protect your plants from wind, rain, and harsh sun. If you don't have a greenhouse, you can start your seeds outside on a table, but you'll need to pull them back inside during a hard rain.

Water your seeds twice a day, giving them a thorough soak with a Fogg-It nozzle.

If you're going to use an existing Crop Garden, Bulletproof Garden, or raised beds for your winter planting, go ahead and finish harvesting from those beds. Don't worry about small weeds, since they'll be killed with the silage tarp later on. Do add compost or any amendments you want in the soil to give things time to settle before planting.

Also, bugs can be intense during the end of summer, so it's probably a good idea to cover your starts with a bug net. Just hang the net on top of your soil blocks. Your plants will lift it up with them as they grow.

Three weeks before planting. If you haven't built beds in your garden area yet, now's the time. To do that, shovel from what will be a flat footpath (about 12 inches wide) and put the dirt on your bed. Usually our beds range from 2 to 4 inches tall. To ensure a straight bed, set up a string line by driving a post at either end of the bed and hanging a string between the posts to guide you as you dig.

Once your beds are ready, put down your silage tarp to kill off any remaining vegetation. Then water down the garden area before you put down the tarp. The water will encourage worm activity and will go a long way toward getting everything broken down and ready for you to plant in just a few weeks. Having silage tarps over the area will also prevent weed growth until you are ready to transplant your seed starts.

Last, figure out how many low tunnels you will require. Remember, one low tunnel will cover two garden beds that are 30 inches wide and 50 feet long, with a 12-inch path in between. Order your supplies for those tunnels.

One week before planting. Begin hardening off your seed starts. The first half of the week, bring them outside for half the day. Then the last half of the week, bring them outside all day. Hardening off your plants

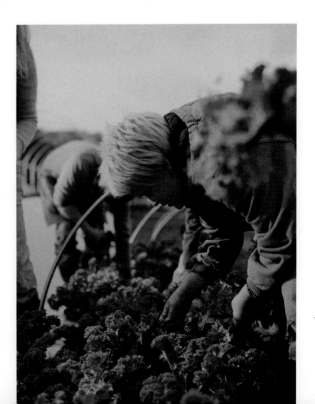

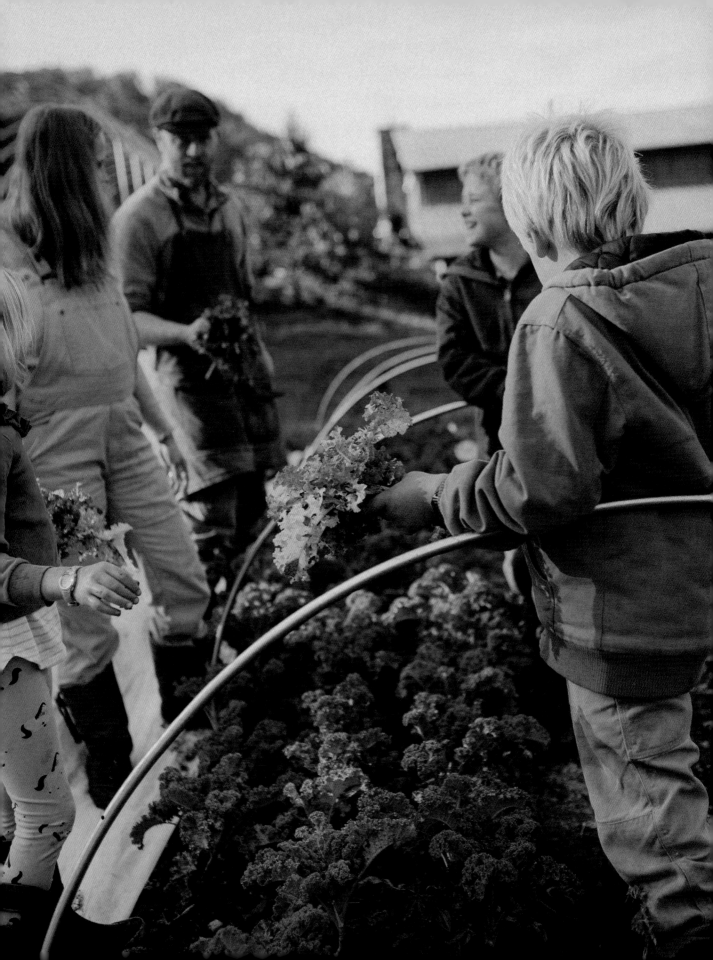

gradually gets them ready for the big world by exposing them to the wind and direct sun. The soil blocks will literally get harder as they are exposed to more elements. In the event of heavy rain, however, be sure to bring your plants in so as not to destroy their soil blocks.

Planting. Remove your silage tarp from the garden and transplant your starts. Add your low tunnel framing and get your weights in place so you're ready for the first frost. But don't actually cover the plants until that first frost is predicted.

First frost. When the weather forecast says frost is coming, cover your beds with the Agribon cover to complete your low tunnels. Keep it covered every night when frost is possible.

Ventilate. Once the Agribon is in place, you'll need to remove it every day that the temperature rises above 60°F. The easiest way to ventilate is to pull the weights away from one side of the tunnel, and then pull back your Agribon cover. Whenever there's a chance for frost at night, you'll need to put the cover back in place.

Note: Agribon covering is fragile, so be gentle whenever you pull it on or off. Don't worry if you get a few tears or holes. Just plan on replacing the coverings every year.

First snow. The first time there's a threat of snow, add the greenhouse plastic to the Agribon cover. If you get a big snow, over 6 inches, I would recommend taking a broom and sweeping it off to avoid the plastic collapsing. Once again, remove the plastic and the Agribon any time the temperature goes above 60.

———————

There you have it! That's how to build and maintain your Winter Harvest Garden. When done right, this system is an absolute joy. Given that you can have fresh greens all winter without the hassle of weeding or fighting bugs, it's a no-brainer. All you have to do is motivate yourself to get out there and plant when everybody else is wrapping it up for the season, then help those plants get to maturity—a little weeding in the fall and maybe some simple pest control. When the first cold snap comes through, you're pretty much done except for covering and uncovering those tunnels when necessary.

Sure, your neighbors might laugh when they see you planting in August. But you'll be the one laughing all the way to the bank when they see you harvesting greens for Christmas dinner from under the snow!

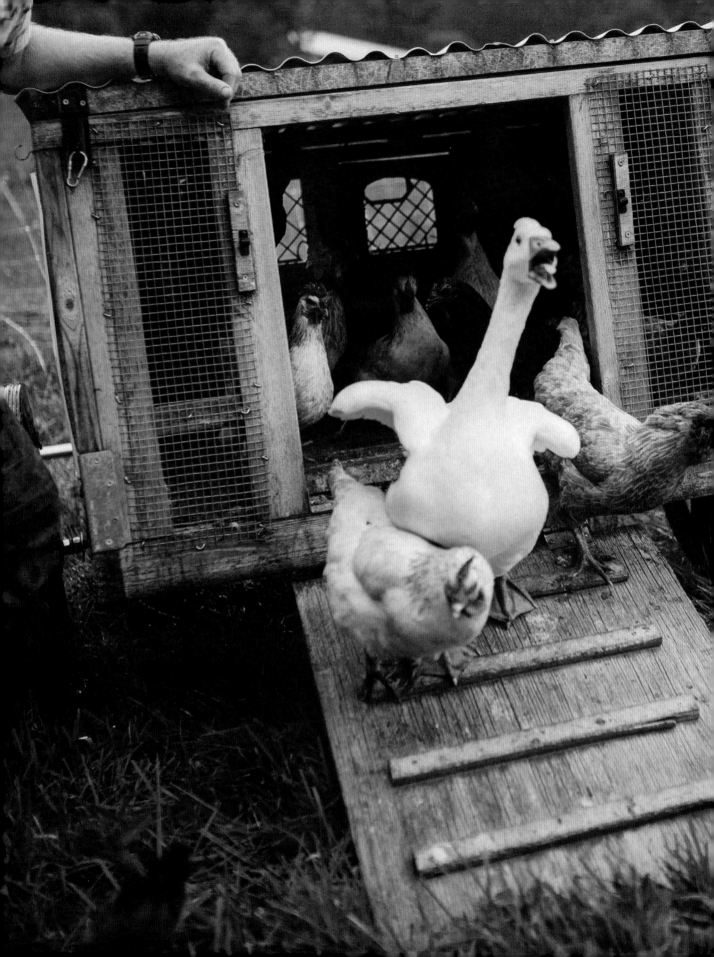

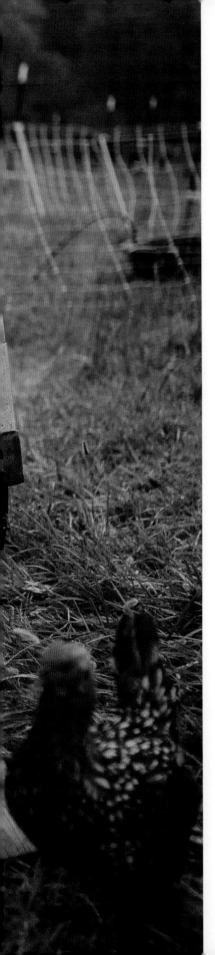

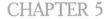

CHAPTER 5

Raising Chickens for Eggs

It was snowing outside, but I was warm and cozy cooking breakfast in our kitchen. I was making my signature dish: bacon-in eggs.

As always, I got started by plopping some bacon (raised on our own homestead) in a cast-iron skillet and letting it start to fry. I waited until there was a little grease in the pan, then I chopped up the bacon into bite-size pieces. Then, I was ready to add the eggs for scrambling.

Is your mouth watering yet? It should be. My signature eggs are that good.

There was just one problem that particular morning: no eggs! I looked over at the spot on our counter where we usually keep the previous day's harvest, but it was empty. The kids must have had a hankering for hard-boiled eggs the night before.

What to do? I ran outside in my boxer shorts and T-shirt. (That's what I wear when I make breakfast, y'all.) I zipped down the garden path, thankful that the snowy weather was keeping the public road next to our house pretty much unoccupied. As I hoped, I found several eggs ready to go in the chicken coop no more than 100 feet from my door. The cold was really starting to prickle on my feet and legs, but I used the bottom of my shirt

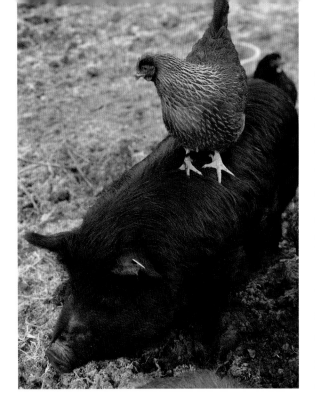

as an impromptu basket and scooped up all the eggs I could find—then rushed back inside.

Just in time! The bacon was perfect, the grease was ready, and I cracked those eggs like a whiz to start the scramble. Delicious.

People tell me all the time that growing your own food sounds hard. Well, it is in some ways. But rushing out to the grocery store every time you need something for a meal is hard too. So is working a job to get money to pay the bill at that store. And so is dealing with unnecessary medical trouble when all the unhealthy food you've eaten comes back to haunt you.

When my family needs eggs, we typically walk over to the counter and find fresh, organic eggs harvested just twelve hours before. When we're hungry for a salad, we grab some greens from our gardens—even in the dead of winter with snow on the ground. When we need bacon or are itching for a burger, we walk to one of our freezers and cook up meat we raised ourselves with no steroids, no hormones, no chemicals of any kind.

That is the hidden power of the rooted life. Yes, we eat healthier than we ever could from the store. And yes, we're saving money. But on top of that, there is nothing more convenient

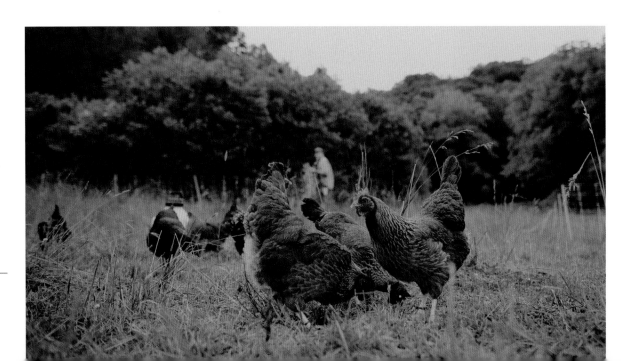

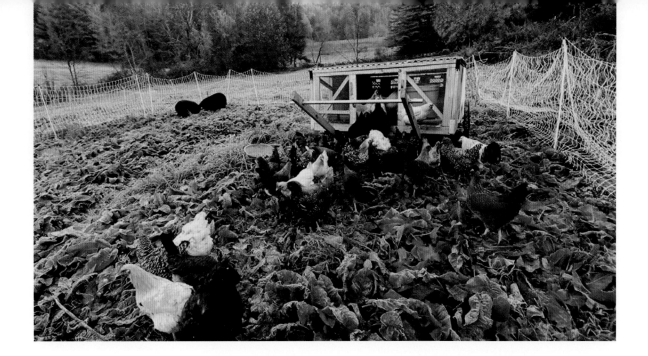

than just walking out your front door for a fresh, healthy meal.

So far in these pages we've focused mainly on gardening and growing produce, which is a great first step. And I want to say this again: if that's the only step you take—if gardening is all you have room for in terms of your time, your land, or your heart—that's okay. In fact, that's great! You are contributing to your family's health and wellness by growing a significant portion of your own food, which is a wonderful goal.

But if you're ready to take the next step by maximizing what you grow and adding fresh eggs and fresh meat to your family's table, then chickens are the way to go. And I'm excited to show you how to get started!

Learning the Basics

If the idea of raising chickens sounds scary, I understand. It's definitely a different experience, and it is a higher level of commitment than growing vegetables. But as I hope to show you over the next few chapters, the benefits are exponential—and not just in terms of eggs and meat. Chickens will be the hardest workers in your gardens as well. They'll till the land, debug not just your gardens but your entire yard, provide great compost, and much more. (We'll dig deeper into the sweet synergy between chickens and gardens in Chapter 7.)

All that being said, let's cover the basics by addressing some of the questions I receive most often about raising chickens.

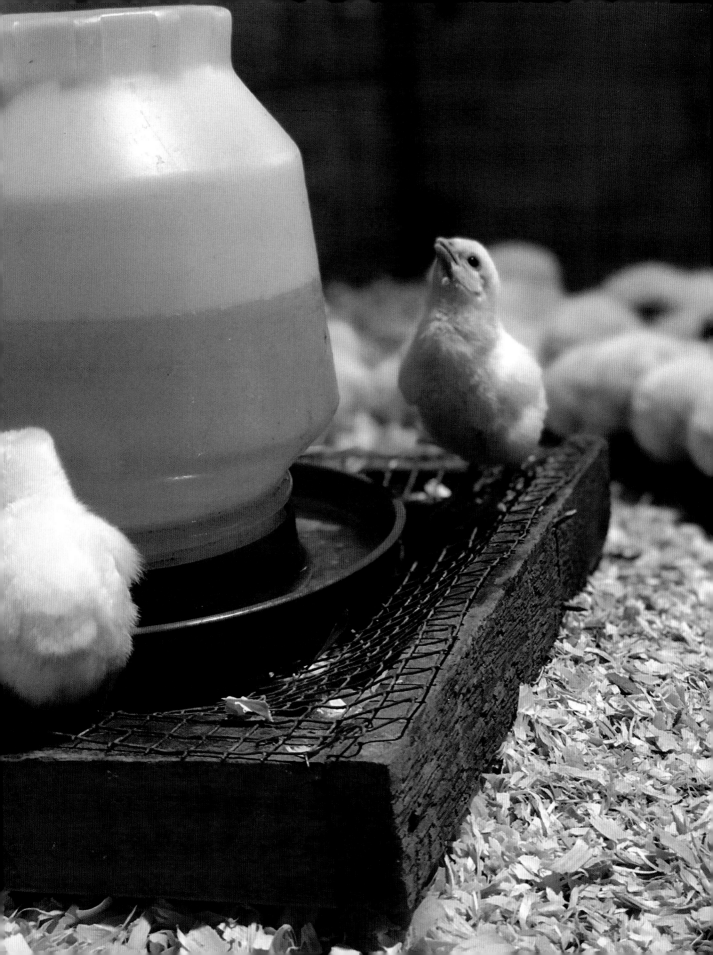

What structures do I need to set up?

If you're going to grow your chickens from chicks—which is what I recommend and which is the method I'll offer instructions for below—you'll need to start with a brooder. A brooder is a contained space where your chicks can eat, drink, and sleep protected against the outside world while they are still young. It's like a nursery for chicks.

Once the chickens are old enough to be outside, you'll need two more elements. The first is a place for them to sleep, which is usually called a coop or a chicken house. The second is a chicken run, pasture, or other fenced area where they can do what chickens do during the daylight hours—peck, scratch, hunt for bugs, socialize, and so on.

That's it! Of course, there are lots of different options and designs out there for how to set up your chickens, but I'm going to offer three systems later in this chapter that work great and are easy to both set up and maintain.

Does it stink?

This is the question I'm asked most often about raising chickens, and the answer is a big, fat no! Frankly, any bad smell on a homestead is a symptom of bad management, and that's definitely the case with chickens. They don't have to stink.

The best way to manage the smell and mess that chickens *can* produce is by using deep bedding or by moving them regularly. Deep bedding is any kind of natural material you use to cover the ground in your chicken coop and chicken run—wherever chickens are hanging out for long periods of time. These materials can include leaves, organic straw, dry grass clippings, unsprayed hay, or sawdust; or, if you need to purchase something, wood shavings are easy to come by and relatively inexpensive. I like wood chips best because they work great and I can source them from my own land. Plan on starting with at least 4 inches, although 8 inches is ideal.

The idea with deep bedding is that the chickens will do their business on the top layer of the bedding. (Fun fact: Chickens don't pee. They deposit little packets that contain both urine and fecal matter.) Then, in just a little time, the chicken waste filters down to the lower layers of the bedding. Eventually, the bottom layer of your deep bedding will turn into compost, which is great for your gardens.

If you ever do start to notice a smell around your chickens, just add another light layer of deep bedding and walk away. No more smell.

How much work does it require to raise chickens?

Like most things, it takes a little work on the front end to get yourself started with chickens. But once you get your system rolling, it's not a big deal. Here are the basic things you'll need to cover in any given day:

- Let the chickens out each morning.
- Provide food and water.
- If you don't have a permanent chicken coop, move your mobile coop to a new spot, or move your fences if you're pasturing the chickens (more on both of those options below).
- Harvest eggs.
- Put the chickens up for the night.

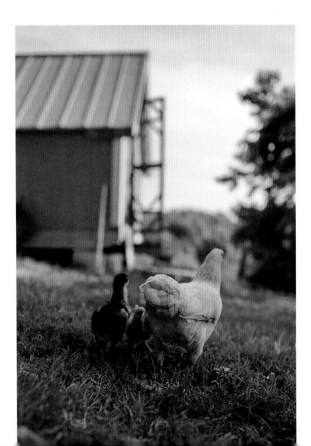

Because we like efficiency in the Rhodes family, we put out food and water when we let the chickens out in the morning, and we move our mobile coops at the same time. Then, we harvest the eggs right before we put the chickens up at night. So, we only have to mess with the chickens twice a day. Easy-peasy.

Am I allowed to raise chickens?

This is something you'll need to determine based on the legal restrictions connected to your situation. Many neighborhoods or HOAs allow chickens but not roosters (which are not necessary anyway); some provide specific limits to the number of birds you can raise. I'm a "It's better to beg for forgiveness than ask for permission" kind of guy, but you'll need to decide for yourself. I do know that giving a few eggs to your neighbors (especially the ornery ones) can go a long way toward keeping them from complaining to the authorities.

If chickens are against the rules in your area, or even the law, there's still hope. There are creative loopholes and ways to change those laws if needed. Should you be one to shake up the system, I highly suggest you check out one of my original chicken mentors, Patricia "Pat" Foreman. I highly recommend her book, *City Chicks*.

Before You Start

I know you're getting excited about those fresh eggs. Can you taste them yet?

Speaking of eggs, the first thing you need to decide is how many chickens you want to raise. And the best way to decide how many chickens to raise is to figure out how many eggs your family will need each week. Your typical egg-laying chicken breed will produce three or four eggs a week—probably more in spring and less in winter, but that's an average.

So, let's say your family needs a dozen eggs a week. That means at the very minimum you would want to raise three or four chickens. If you're like the Rhodes clan and you use a dozen eggs or more every day, you're talking about a minimum of twenty-four lovely ladies to produce enough supply for that demand.

Now, those are textbook numbers, and we all know textbook numbers don't always match with real life. Just like gardening, I recommend you plan to produce 25 percent more than you think you'll need. That's because egg counts will fluctuate, a child will break an egg or two, or maybe one of your birds will get snatched by a predator. Those things happen, so it's best to plan for them now and reduce your stress later.

So, if you think you need only three chickens, plan to raise four. If you think twenty-four is the right number, plan for thirty. You can thank me later.

Here's another fun fact: You do *not* need a rooster to get eggs. A hen (female adult chicken) is happy to produce (unfertilized) eggs without a male. Yes, a male may complete the social structure—I recommend one rooster per fifteen hens—and offer a little bit of protection, but it isn't necessary unless you want to breed your own chickens. Otherwise, everyone will do just fine without him. (I see a lot of ladies nodding their heads as they read this.)

The next thing you need to decide is what kind of chickens you want to raise. I strongly recommend what are called dual-purpose breeds, since they provide eggs but are also good for eating once their egg-laying days are over. Dual birds put out a lot of eggs, thrive in almost any environment, and love to work.

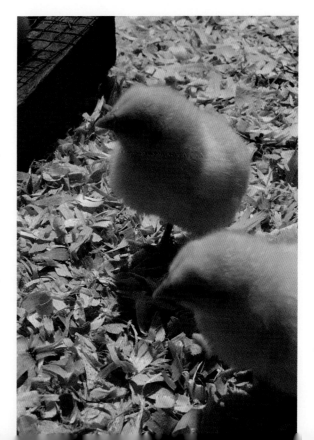

For that reason, I'd recommend any of the following breeds: Rhode Island Red, Barred Plymouth Rock, Black Australorp, Wyandotte, or Buff Orpington. These and other breeds can easily be sourced locally from Craigslist or from an online hatchery such as Murray McMurray, which is where we get our chicks.

Yet another fun fact: Chickens lay eggs in different colors, and you can choose which colors you want when you place your order. My Rebekah really likes a colorful egg basket—a nice rainbow of white, light brown, dark brown, blues, and greens. So, keep that in mind as you order your birds.

Okay, what about timing? I highly recommend getting chicks when nature does: in the spring. That way your little ones have plenty of fresh greens and warm sunshine as they grow up. Specifically, you want to order your chicks so they arrive no more than three weeks before your last possible frost date. Those little chicks will have already grown their feathers and will be ready to graduate from the brooder after three weeks.

Plus, if you get them by spring, they will begin to lay eggs between five and ten months later, which is going into the fall. Then, two years after that, when you go to harvest your old ladies—because their egg production drops in half after two years—you can harvest in the fall and have another batch of chicks coming of age and starting to lay right at the same time.

If it's already too late for you to start chicks in the spring and you don't feel like waiting around until next year, search Craigslist or a similar site for what are called "pullets." These are young chickens others have already raised from chicks. (They're chicken teenagers, basically.) If you can't get pullets, you'll need to sit tight until next year and maybe focus on a Winter Harvest Garden. With chicks, I've found it's best to work with nature rather than against her.

Also, make sure you do *not* get vaccinated chicks. And you may have to request that specifically. Vaccines are largely a product of the conventional poultry industry, where extra interventions are often necessary to keep chicks alive. However, in your situation, where your chickens will get plenty of room plus access to sunshine, fresh air, and greens, vaccines are totally unnecessary.

The drawbacks for using vaccines and medicated feed (see below) are not only that it's an unnecessary expense and procedure, it's also adding mysterious chemicals and additives. I'm especially concerned about these additions since I'll be feeding these eggs and meat to my family. Remember, if you are what you eat, then you are also what your food eats!

Furthermore, animals have a natural immunity and should be able to thrive in a healthy environment. Aid given unnecessarily tampers with their natural ability to cope with germs and other troubles, which means they can be in danger of becoming immunodeficient.

Finally, many of the vaccines given to

animals include warnings *not* to consume those animals for fifteen to sixty days after applying. That certainly rules out using them on meat birds, who have a fifty-eight-day life cycle before harvest. And that also makes me wonder why the chemicals would all of a sudden be fit for consumption after just sixty days. Did the harm just dissipate somehow?

For Rebekah and me, the benefits of vaccinated chicks are simply not worth the risk.

What You'll Need

No matter what type of chickens you choose or how many eggs you plan to enjoy, if you're going to start your chicken adventures by raising chicks, you're going to need a brooder. So, here is a basic supply list to help make that happen:

- *Brooding room.* This is just a safe, stable place to set up your brooder. We've had brooders in our garage, in barn stalls, in a corner of the dining room, and more. The place doesn't matter as long as it's relatively predator-proof, ideally with not more than a 1-inch space open to the outside.
- *Brooder box.* This is where the chicks will actually stay. My preference is to build a wooden box that is 36 inches tall. Internally, you need 1 square foot for every four chicks to give them enough space. You can also use one or more large plastic storage totes if you won't have a lot of chicks.
- *Watering station.* Pick something small that you can easily keep clean. I use something called a "quart jar waterer," which can be found at Tractor Supply or online and fits easily onto a standard quart-size jar—something you probably have in your house already.
- *Feeding station.* You can also get a "quart jar feeder" to match the watering system. Again, choose something small that you can keep clean.
- *Fine pine shavings.* Fill the brooder with 4 to 8 inches of these shavings—you can get them cheap from Tractor Supply.
- *Mess-catch system.* You need something to keep your feeding and watering stations clean of manure and pine shavings. This can be as simple as a piece

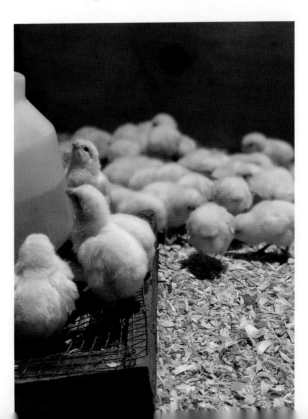

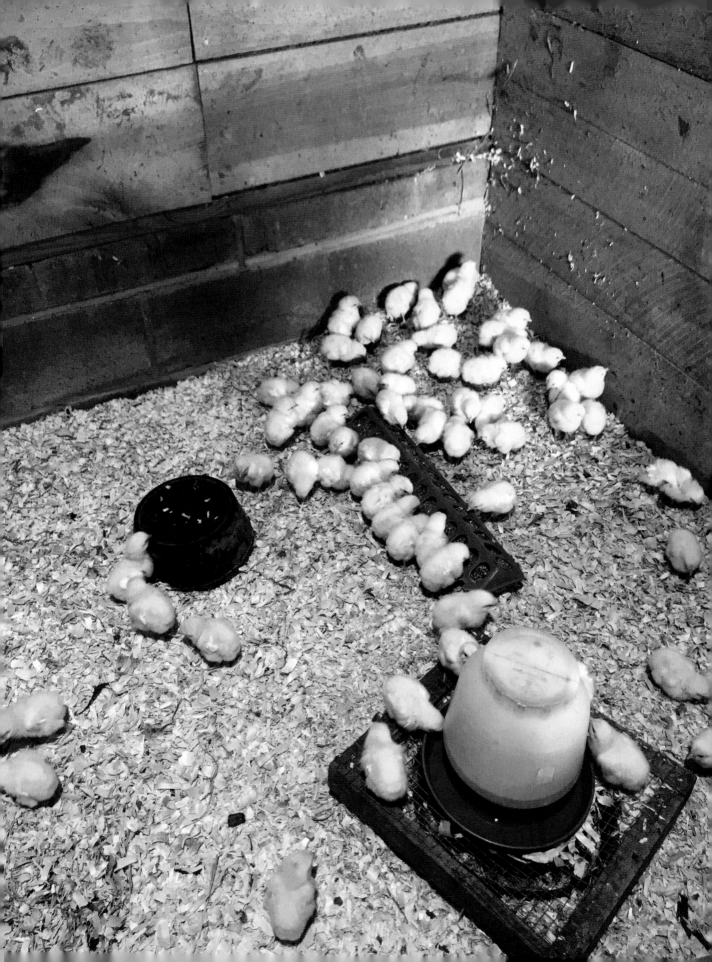

of cardboard laid under the food/water and changed as needed. Or it can be a homemade wooden frame with a piece of ½-inch hardware cloth mounted to it. Make this big enough to hold both the watering station and feeder, and size it to fit over a feed pan buried in the shavings (so that the food and water stay at ground level). You can also purchase a chick stand from Premier 1.

- *Warmth.* Your new chicks' first desire will be to get warm. Warmth, water, and then food. I really like Premier 1's Heating Plates, which I call "hoverers." They come in four different sizes to accommodate different sizes of brooders and flocks. The hoverers act more like a natural mother and don't put off any light.

If you're short on space and/or dollar bills, you can go with a heat lamp and a 150-watt red heat bulb. We use a combination of lamp and hoverer in our large brooder. We put the lamp over the feeding station to keep the food warm, and the hoverer for the chicks to hang out underneath.

Once your brooder is ready to go, you'll also need what I call *rooster teeth* for your chicks. (Normal people just call it "grit," but that's no fun.) Chickens don't have teeth, so they grind their food by swallowing small rocks that end up in their gizzards—a muscle pouch where their food gets ground up. I prefer using creek sand because it has more minerals, but you can also buy grit from a supply store.

And, of course, you'll need feed for your chicks. Begin with chick or poultry starter feed. It's high in protein and ground down nicely for your little birds. Count on each chick eating 1½ to 2 pounds of feed for the first three to four weeks. You can keep them on starter feed indefinitely or switch to grower feed once they're eight weeks old (this may be a little more affordable).

This is important: *Do not* get medicated feed. Why? Because, like vaccines, it's not necessary for your home-raised chicken posse with access to fresh air, occasional greens, and plenty of sunshine. And seriously, if you read the ingredients label on a bag of medicated feed, you'd need a medical degree to understand all the words there. It's never made sense for me to feed my animals chemicals I have to look up on Google to understand—especially when there are simple, organic, and non-GMO feeds out there with a readable and understandable ingredient list of corn, peas, wheat, fish meal, and so on. Rebekah and I have used New Country Organics for years. You might be able to find this brand (or request it) at your local farm or garden store, or you can have it shipped to your front door.

Last, you'll need a system to house and maintain your chickens once they're out of the brooder and ready for their journey toward egg-laying glory. Thankfully, the three systems I like best are all easy to set up and easy to maintain. You can find detailed supply lists and building instructions (with lots of pictures!) for all three of these systems at TheRootedLife .com/Resources.

Option 1: The Compost Corner

Most backyard or homestead chickens are kept in what's called a static run. Meaning, they have a coop and a fence that stays in the same place all the time. This in and of itself is not a bad thing—*if* you honor spacing requirements and incorporate deep bedding (what my mentor Joel Salatin calls a "carbonaceous diaper").

Sadly, what usually happens in these chicken runs is something rather nasty. The birds end up scratching and pooping in the same area over and over again until you've got a manure-icing moonscape that's absolutely disgusting and incredibly smelly. No wonder the neighbors are complaining and folks are making rules against these birds.

Fortunately, there's a much better way to set up a static chicken system—one that stays in the same place all the time but doesn't stink and is easy to maintain. Even better, this system produces valuable compost for your garden, which is why I call it the Compost Corner.

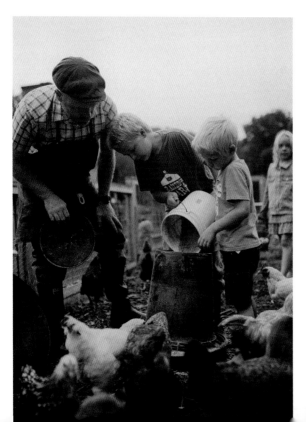

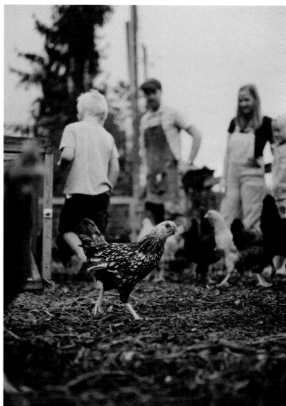

You should consider a Compost Corner if you:

- Already have a stationary chicken coop and run (a fenced-in area) you want to keep using and/or improve.
- Want or have a permanent garden area (like raised beds) near your chickens so they can complement each other. (More on this excellent idea in Chapter 7.)
- Want a low-maintenance system throughout the year, but you can handle a few hard hours putting in deep bedding and harvesting compost (more on the latter in Chapter 7).
- Have enough space to dedicate 3 square feet per bird in their chicken run, and 9 inches of perch space in the coop—with the perches placed 12 inches apart. That means four birds would need 12 square feet of space. Thirty chickens? About 150 square feet.

To set up a Compost Corner, you'll start with a chicken coop, which can be permanent or mobile. Then you'll add fencing around the coop to keep the chickens in and predators out—remember, at least 3 square feet for every bird. This is your chicken run. Then you fill the whole area with 4 to 8 inches of deep bedding.

All that's left is food and water. For food, you can toss the chicken feed directly on the ground, which will encourage your birds to scratch and peck around the deep bedding.

Or you can use a feeder. If you do use a feeder, make sure it's set up off the bedding. I use a non-pressure-treated pallet to set out my food and water; this is great because the birds have to hop up out of the mulch to get their food, which keeps things cleaner.

For water, I recommend a 1-, 3-, or 5-gallon vacuum-sealed waterer. We like the Little Giant brand. Four chickens will drink 1 quart of water a day. I recommend you provide at least enough water for a day so you're doing that chore only once. You could also get a large enough waterer to change it every three days. Any longer than three days is not good because the water can get nasty.

I do want to offer one word about fencing. I recommend you start with temporary fences, such as Premier 1's electric netting. That's because you can never be quite sure the fence is in the right place when you're getting started—you may want to move things around and experiment. Once you've had a temporary fence in the same place for three years, it's probably safe to build something permanent.

And that's it! That's all it takes to create a stable, productive, easy-to-maintain system for your lovely egg-laying ladies.

Reminder: You can find free plans for building a Compost Corner at TheRootedLife .com/Resources.

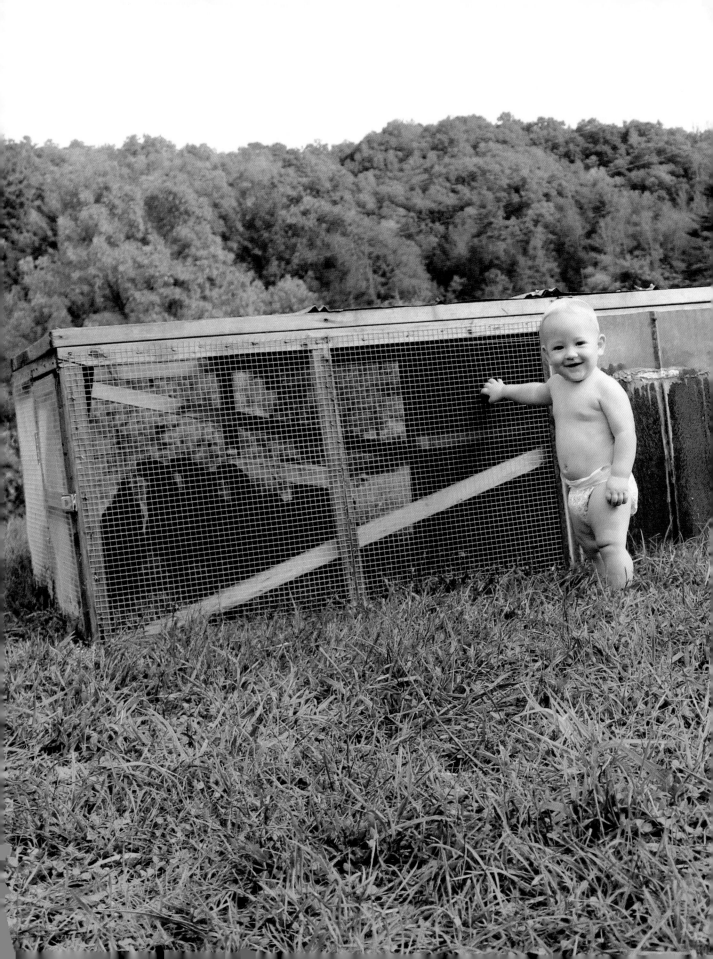

Option 2: The Chicken Tractor

In my mind, this is the simplest way to keep a small number of chickens in your yard, yet it's also powerful. I call this system the Chicken Tractor because it doesn't just keep your chickens alive and give them a place to lay eggs—it puts them to work. It harnesses the power of chickens doing what chickens do: scratching, tilling, and fertilizing your lawns or gardens.

This system is designed to serve as the chickens' coop, fence, and run all at the same time, and it's incredibly simple. As you can see from the pictures, the idea is to create a rectangular box that houses the chickens' nesting areas and allows them to be protected at night. But it also gives the chickens space to run around on the ground and enjoy fresh greens from your yard.

Most important, the Chicken Tractor is mobile. Rather than stay in one place, it's designed to be moved to a new location in your yard or garden each day. That way the chickens can spread their pecking, scratching, and fertilizing magic all over your property. (As you'll see in Chapter 7, this can also work especially well for preparing the ground for gardens.)

In terms of numbers, my Chicken Tractor is designed to house four egg-layers or twenty meat chickens. It also includes an optional door for more flexibility. If you want to open things up in the afternoon, you can allow your chickens to free-range around the yard, debugging the grass or other crops while finding free food for themselves. (You can also use temporary nets to keep the chickens

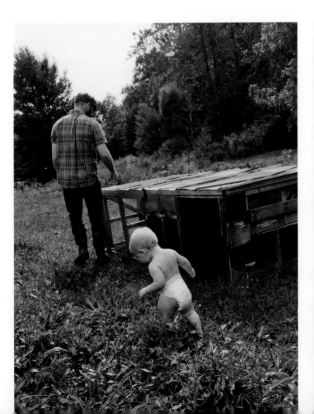
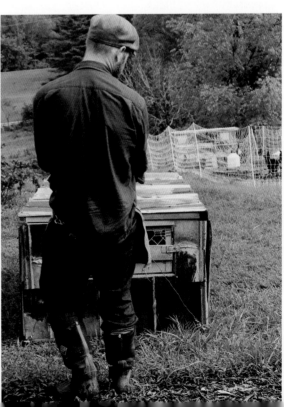

in specific areas and protect them from predators.) This makes the Chicken Tractor into a "hen hotel" for as many as twelve birds.

You should consider using the Chicken Tractor as your primary chicken system if you:

- Don't have a lot of space.
- Just want to keep a few chickens (fewer than twelve).
- Want the extra health benefit of pasture-raised eggs. (When chickens have fresh greens and space to run, their eggs are more nutritious.)
- Need a low-profile setup that doesn't look like a chicken operation.
- Can afford the roughly $350 in start-up costs.

Reminder: You can find free plans for building a Chicken Tractor at TheRootedLife .com/Resources.

Option 3: The Yard/Pasture

Joel Salatin, one of my mentors, has made a huge mark on the organic-growing and homesteading movements of recent decades. Joel has always been a big proponent of keeping chickens mobile in order to let them work the land, and then allowing the sun to sanitize that same area once the chickens move on.

Joel's method for this movement is what he calls an "Egg Mobile," which is a large coop (sometimes two) on wheels that can be hooked to a tractor and moved around the farm. I knew I wanted to do this during my early days of raising chickens, but I didn't have a tractor and I didn't want or need hundreds of birds. I was pondering how to move a small flock of chickens by hand when I happened to see a concept Eliot Coleman dreamed up in *The New Organic Grower*. He called it the "ChickShaw"

because it was inspired by an Asian rickshaw, which makes a heavy load easy enough for a single person to move. Without getting into the physics, centering the weight over two wheels makes the load easy to pull at one end.

The only problem with Eliot's concept was that it was made out of metal electrical conduit or similar materials, which means it needed to be fabricated. That got me to put on my thinking cap. Could this thing be made out of material that ordinary folks can access and use? Eventually I got to work on my own ChickShaw design. Now, after several improvements, my ChickShaw really does make moving chickens around the small homestead quite easy.

At the core, my ChickShaw carries out the same function as the Chicken Tractor, just scaled up to handle more birds. It can handle and house up to thirty egg-laying chickens or ninety meat chickens. That's a lot of food-producing poultry!

You should consider using the ChickShaw as your chicken system if you:

- Want a larger flock of feathered friends.
- Want the extra health benefit of pasture-raised eggs.
- Want to fertilize a larger yard or small pasture by moving your chickens around weekly.
- Have a good amount of yard or pasture to give the chickens a weekly rotation without returning to the starting point for three to ten weeks (depending on how long the grass takes to recover).
- Want an easily maintained day-to-day operation but are able to move the coop and electric net once a week.

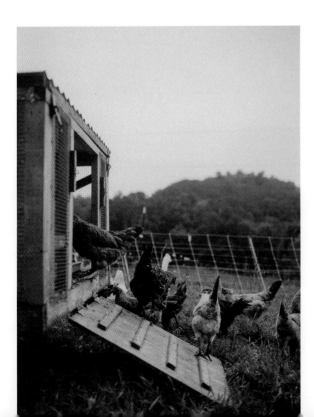

- Are willing to keep the coop and net in one spot over the winter on deep bedding or a future garden plot.
- Can afford roughly $1,500 in start-up supplies.

What You'll Need

Reminder: You can find free plans for building a ChickShaw at TheRootedLife.com/Resources.

- My ChickShaw Mini-Me (12–30 chickens) or my ChickShaw (24–60 chickens).
- 5-gallon vacuum-sealed waterer.
- Feeder (optional). I just throw their feed on the ground to encourage scratching.
- I like the 48-inch-tall nets from Premier 1 as they help prevent the chickens from jumping over the top. I recommend 100 feet of fence for twelve-ish chickens. Use 164 feet of fence (roughly 1,200 square feet) for up to 30–60 chickens. But if you struggle with the strength, you could opt for shorter nets in height and length. Net sizes go down to 30-ish inches and come in as little as 50-foot lengths.
- Solar energizer kit (includes tester and grounding rod). I like Premier 1 energizers, and I recommend something with as many joules as you can afford and still be able to carry.

How to Make It Happen

"Hello?" The first time we received new chicks in the mail, the post office called at 4:30 in the morning. I didn't want the clerk to think I was a slacker, so I pretended to be awake (and cheerful) when I said, "This is Justin."

"Your chicks are ready to be picked up." He didn't sound very awake either. But I did hear a lot of chirping in the background.

I was out the door in just a few minutes. I knew the chicks had traveled a long way, and I wanted to pick them up ASAP. I did turn on the heat in my brooder before I left, though. Chicks want to be warm even before they look for food and water, and I wanted everything to be ready when we got back to the house. I also asked Rebekah to prepare a one-time batch of "Magic Water" while I was gone. That's 1 gallon of warm water, ½ cup of honey, ¼ cup of apple cider vinegar (we like Bragg's), and 4 minced garlic cloves.

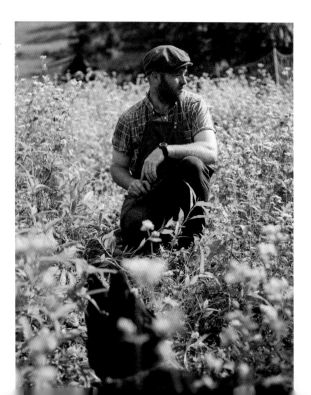

You might not get a call before dawn on the day your chicks arrive, but you still need to be ready to give them a head start on their health. So, I'll finish up this chapter by giving you a detailed timeline of what you can expect—and what you need to do—to raise your egg-laying chickens from their first day with you until their last.

Day one. When you first bring the chicks home, remove them from the shipping crate one at a time. Dip their beaks into the Magic Water for an immune-system boost and set them in the warm brooder. Don't be surprised if a couple of chicks died during their shipping journey. (And don't be surprised if the hatchery sent extra for that very reason.)

Fill your feeding and watering stations, this time with plain water, and make sure that at least a third of your chicks can access the food at the same time. Also add rooster teeth (grit) in a small feed pan.

If you can, gather some green grass, lettuce, kale, or other green foods, shred it by hand, and add it to your brooder. The chlorophyll in the greens will go a long way toward keeping the chicks healthy.

First two weeks. It's best practice to check on your chicks twice a day as long as they're in the brooder. They'll eat and poop very little at first, so don't be alarmed. It's important they have access to food and water 24-7. Fill and/or clean out waterers and feeders as needed. Fresh grass clippings or similar greens are great to add every day. Continue to add garden produce or food scraps as a supplement to the feed.

During the third week. Start "hardening off" the chicks. This is the process of weaning these little ones off their heat and preparing them for the world. Start by turning off their heat source during the day. Then, about the middle of that third week, turn off the heat lamps completely, even at night. This will help them transition to the temperatures outside.

After three weeks. Move your chicks to their outside coop. *Important:* Do this in the evening. Allowing them to spend the night in the coop will teach the chicks where their new home is, especially if you have other chickens in the coop. And, yes it's fine to introduce young chicks to an older flock (even if you have roosters). It's totally natural for chickens of various ages to be together.

If you've got freezing temperatures at night, it's okay to wait a little longer to bring the chicks out into the cold—up to four or even six weeks. Just be sure to add enough bedding in the brooder to deal with their manure load.

Once the chicks are in their coop, set out a grit/mineral feeder and fill it with grit, kelp (we use Thorvin), and aragonite. (Premier 1 makes a grit feeder for dispensing this.) Kelp is full of essential vitamins and trace minerals that help boost the chicks' immune systems, strengthen the shells of their eggs, offer bone support, and help make their egg yolks

orange. Aragonite is a form of calcium that also supports their bones, enhances egg production, and increases feed consumption efficiency (more weight gain with less food). Have grit, kelp, and aragonite available for the chicks to eat whenever they choose, but don't be surprised if their demand ebbs and flows.

Next, set up a dust bath—just an open box that is halfway filled with dirt. Chickens don't like showers or baths to stay clean, but they love to wallow in the dirt. They have an oil gland on their tails they use for preening, and they'll jump into the dust bath to keep mites and other small critters at bay.

Three weeks to five months. Keep feeding your chicks all they can eat until they're eating more than ⅓ pound (dry weight) of feed per day, per bird. Once they hit that mark, begin rationing their feed to that amount. For example, twelve adult chickens should eat 4 pounds of feed a day. If given the choice, your chickens will eat too much food, which is not good for them—an overweight hen will lay fewer eggs.

At eight weeks. Finish up whatever starter feed you have left and switch to grower feed. It's coarser, making it more efficient. The starter feed is more powdery, which can make it difficult for chickens to eat as they continue to grow.

Five to ten months. Expect your first egg anywhere during this period. (And be ready for some excitement when it comes!) Once you get your first egg, you can finish up your grower feed and switch to layer feed.

A year and a half. Toward the fall of the year, don't be surprised if your chickens start to lose their feathers and drop their egg production. If they're older than a year, they're going through what is called a molt. This is when they'll lose old feathers and grow new ones. To keep everyone healthy, feed them crushed eggshells, kelp, and aragonite on demand.

Two years. If you want to keep egg production as efficient as possible, this is the time to order a new batch of chicks. That way the new chicks have enough time to grow up before they replace your older ladies.

Two and a half years. Once your new chickens start to lay eggs, you can cull your old ladies. Now, these may be your beloved friends by this time, and it's fine if you decide to keep them alive. Just know that their egg production will drop in half, but they'll keep eating the same amount.

If you do harvest your older hens, you'll want to plan on slow-cooking them. We've found that the older birds make a great meat stock. Cook them slowly, since they'll be much tougher than the young, tender meat birds you're probably used to eating.

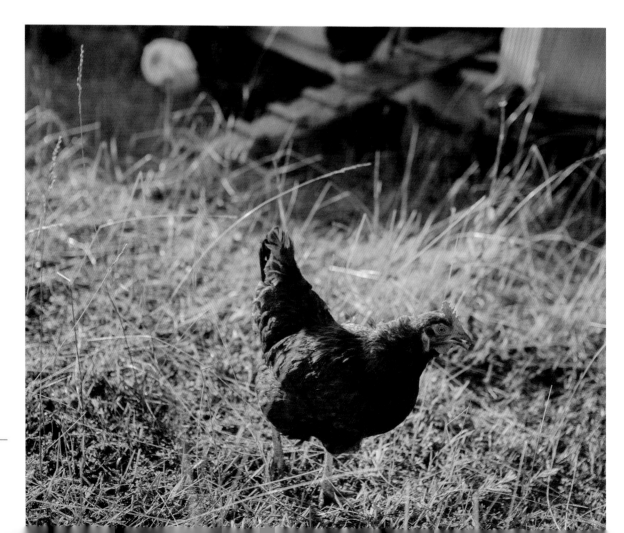

Final Tips and Tricks

As I hope you've seen in this chapter, raising chickens for eggs is not a daunting task. In fact, it often feels like a privilege. Your chickens will be the hardest-working members of your homestead family, and they'll repay your efforts with an abundance of fresh food.

So, here are some final best practices for keeping those helping hens living their best lives each and every day:

- Allow the birds access to their coop or other shelter during the day to serve as shade and extra protection from aerial predators.
- Keep their water as clean as possible. Pat Foreman says you want their water to be clean enough for you to drink. Just don't lose heart if they mess it up within hours (or even minutes). Your best bet is to do a light cleaning once a day and a thorough cleaning once a week with brushes.
- If you like, add 2 tablespoons of organic raw apple cider vinegar (we use Bragg's) per gallon of water in the watering station once a month—or even once a week. This natural health boost will go a long way toward keeping everyone well.
- Feed your chickens food scraps of all kinds. I mean, why throw *any* scrap of food in the trash when you have chickens? They get free food, and they convert your food "waste" into delicious eggs and meat. As I mentioned earlier, it is possible for chickens to eat too much. So, count 2 pounds of food scraps as the equivalent of 1 pound of chicken feed. (Because scraps aren't specifically formulated for chickens the way feed is.)
- Don't feed your chickens junk food. Chickens do a great job of determining what they should and should not eat. Meaning, they won't poison themselves, provided they have other good options for food. Still, don't toss junk food to your birds. Organic moldy cheese? Heck yes. McDonald's hamburger? No way.

Let me finish by saying this: Don't be afraid of chickens. Those glorious birds are hardy and easy to come by. Not only will they provide your family with food generously and consistently, they'll also improve your yard and help manage your gardens.

You really can do this!

Oh, and that first homegrown fried egg? It will be the best you've ever had. Guaranteed.

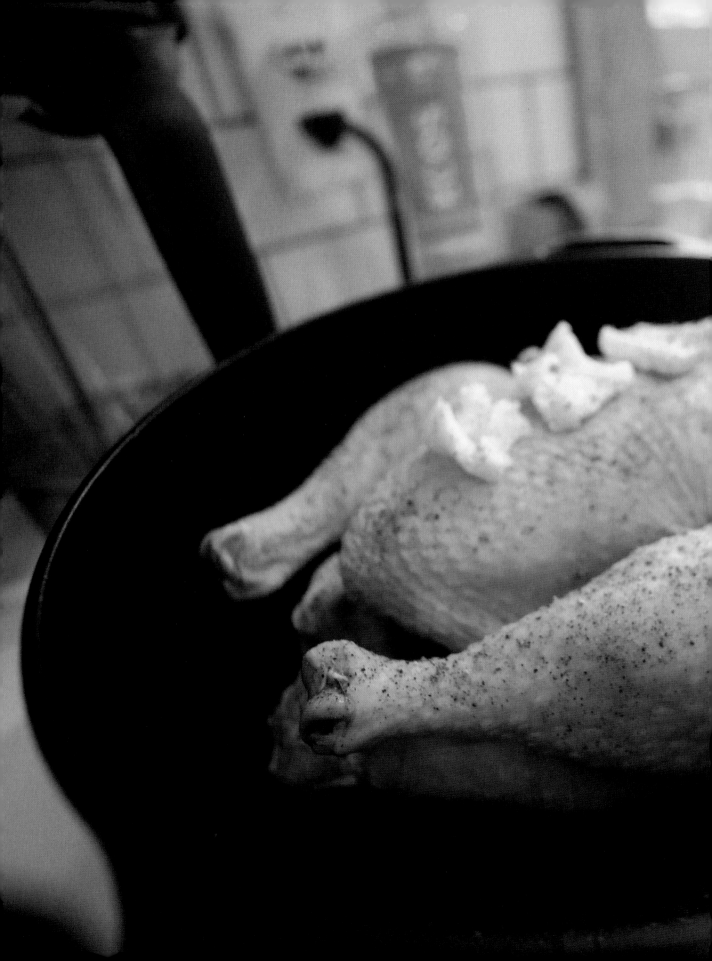

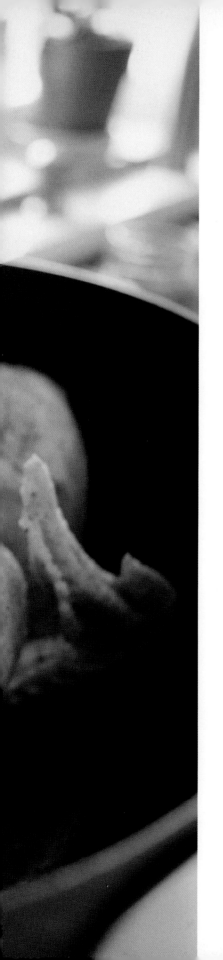

CHAPTER 6

Raising Chickens for Meat

It was harvest day, but I was feeling a little apprehensive. Skeptical, even. This was the first time Rebekah and I had ever raised chickens for meat on our own homestead, and we'd started the venture with a ton of anticipation. But as I looked out across our flock of meat birds, things were looking far less glorious than I'd hoped.

To give you a little background, Rebekah and I decided to spring for "purebred" chickens on our first attempt. These are often called "heritage" birds because they come from a specific breeding stock and are sustainable. When you breed a Rhode Island Red hen with a Rhode Island Red rooster, you get a Rhode Island Red chick. Then, once that chick grows up, it can be bred to produce another Rhode Island Red.

At the time, Rebekah and I weren't planning on breeding our own hens. We were just raising a batch of fifty or so chickens that we planned to harvest for meat. Still, we liked the idea of being sustainable.

So, we ordered our purebreds. Then, we spent the next sixteen weeks taking care of them. It was four months of watering. Four months of feeding—and boy, those heritage birds sure could eat! Four months of moving their mobile pen multiple times a day in the hot sun. Four months of setting out temporary fencing and protecting against predators.

Four months of work, and now the reward was at hand. Or so we hoped. Looking down at those little purebreds, what should have been Christmas Eve felt more like the first day of school.

We got to work harvesting and plucking each bird. They definitely didn't get any bigger after they lost their feathers. Worse, we kept track of each chicken's weight as we worked, and the birds were averaging between 2 and 3 pounds each. Worse still, these heritage birds had practically no breast meat.

You remember those old rubber chicken toys? That's exactly what we were looking at as we plucked and weighed each of our precious purebred birds.

Rebekah and I can laugh now about the moment we plucked that first heritage bird, but we weren't laughing then. It was a deflating experience to say the least.

Introducing the C-Monster

The biggest lesson we learned from that first batch of meat chickens was that the type of chicken matters. A lot.

When we first made the decision to raise meat birds, I used Joel Salatin's classic book *Pastured Poultry Profit* as my guide, scaling it down a bit to a homestead level. I followed Joel's instructions for the brooder. I built a smaller version of his mobile poultry pen. I did everything he said to do—*except* follow his suggestion to raise Cornish Cross meat chickens. I wanted to be a purist. I wanted to be known as "sustainable." So I chose to raise purebred heritage birds instead.

Big mistake, at least in terms of growing our own meat. For eggs? They would absolutely work.

If you're not familiar with the different types of chickens out there, the Cornish Cross meat chicken is what you're used to eating. It's over 4 pounds when it gets to your table, has plenty of breast meat, is tender and juicy, and has a pleasant neutral taste that makes it a favorite main dish or a complementary meat in casseroles, salads, and so on. Cornish Cross is a hybrid breed, meaning it has two types of chickens as parents—a Cornish chicken bred with a White Rock chicken. But it's not genetically modified. It doesn't require steroids or hormones. It's just a specific type of chicken bred to grow quickly and produce a lot of meat.

Oh, and I call them C-monsters for reasons that are probably obvious by now. The "C" is for Cornish and the "monster" is because of their (almost) freakishly fast growth rate.

When Rebekah and I raised our second

batch of meat chickens, we ordered the Cornish Cross. What a difference!

They grew well in the brooder and thrived on daily moves in our pasture pen. (I had to move the heritage birds two or three times a day because they were so active.) The C-monsters drank their water well and ate very efficiently. And boy, did they pack on the pounds! Overall, they were a pleasure to raise. I've been raising these miracle birds for years now, and I have to say that choosing our C-monsters has been one of the best decisions we've made for putting food on our family's table.

To show you what I mean, remember that it took sixteen weeks for those purebred chickens to reach 2 or 3 pounds. C-monsters will reach 4 to 6 pounds freezer weight in just *sixty days*! That means twice the amount of meat in half the time as heritage or dual-purpose birds. And that's without hormones or steroids or special feed of any kind.

Really, the math is hard to beat. If you were to order one hundred Cornish Cross meat chickens, you might expect to lose ten of them during the growing process. (That's normal.) So, after about eight weeks you would be ready to harvest ninety C-monsters at an average of 5 pounds each. That's 450 pounds of food in just sixty days! To give you a comparison, it would take two or three *years* for one cow to give you that much meat. It would take two or three pigs eight to ten months to give you that much meat.

The long and short of it is that C-monsters put food in your freezer at ludicrous speed. And their efficiency will save you some big-time dollar bills in the long run.

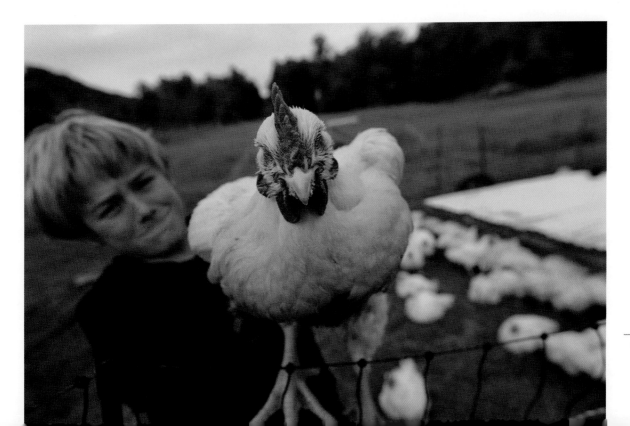

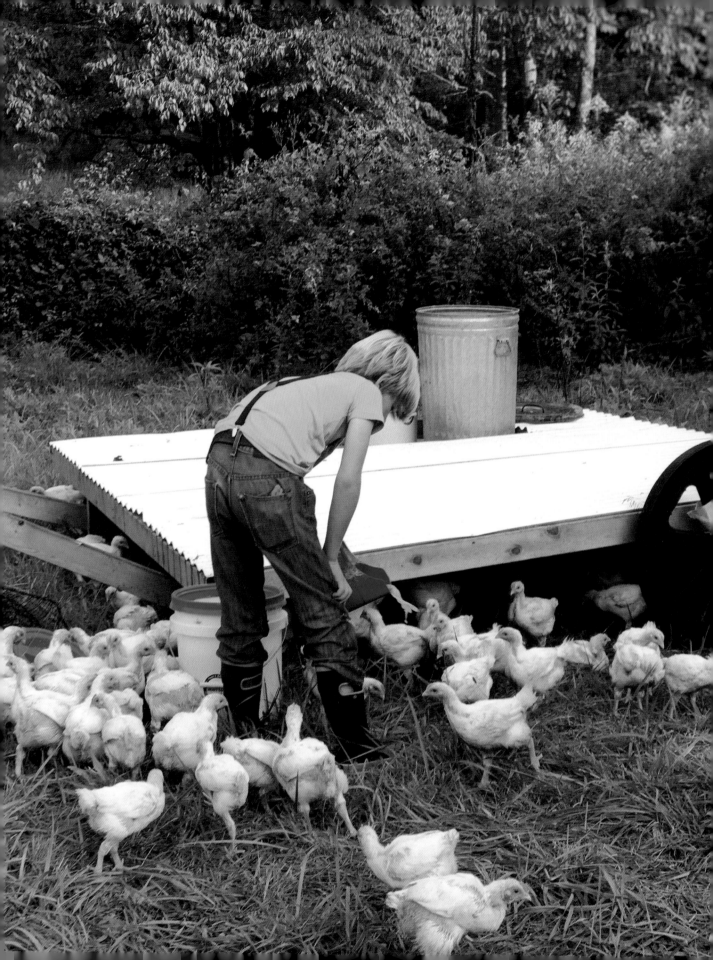

All of this points to the two main reasons why I believe you should consider raising chickens for meat as part of your system for growing your own food. (Assuming you have the space.)

The first reason is food security. If you remember going to the freezer at your local grocery store during the early days of the COVID-19 pandemic and seeing no chicken for sale, you've seen firsthand the dangers of relying on an antiquated supply chain to feed your family. But you don't have to feel that fear again. You can take things into your own hands, and in just two months, you can grow enough meat to cover most or all of your family's needs for an entire year.

The second reason is cost. If you were to buy organic, non-GMO chicken at your local grocery store, you'd likely be spending $6 a pound. And that would be a good investment for the health of your family (compared to buying cheaper birds that are packed with chemicals and never see the light of day).

But by using the system I'll share with you below, you can grow your own organic, non-GMO, *pasture-raised* chicken meat for half that price—just $3 a pound. So, you're saving money and getting better food for your family.

There are lots of other reasons to consider raising chickens for meat. Taste is a big one. So is freshness. And because you'll be feeding your birds real food and letting them out in the sun, your chickens will be packed with nutrients. Besides, this is *chicken* we're talking about! This ain't spinach, although it grows as fast as spinach. This is a food everybody loves. And when you're a part of the story of bringing that food from your own yard to your own table, the experience will be enhanced all the more.

Best of all, you can do this. You don't have to be a pro to raise chickens for meat. You don't have to invest a lot of time or even a lot of space—which is important, because most other meats you raise do require a good bit of land. You just need to be willing to put in some work on the front end and make a little effort each day to raise your birds right for a month and a half. That's it.

Trust me, the rewards will far exceed your investment. Pound for pound, raising meat chickens is one of the most powerful steps you can take in terms of growing your own food. Are you ready?

What You'll Need

The supply lists and instructions below are intended for raising one hundred Cornish Cross meat chickens—which, as a reminder, will produce between 450 and 500 pounds of fresh, organic, pasture-raised meat in your freezer after just sixty days. Now, you can certainly go with fewer chickens if you choose, but you'll need to scale down the supplies accordingly.

Here's what you'll need for the brooder stage:

- 100 unvaccinated Jumbo Cornish Cross chicks (straight run) from McMurray or a similar hatchery.
- Roughly a 4 x 6-foot brooding box for your chicks (four chicks per square foot). I prefer to make the box 36 inches deep to allow for up to 18 inches of deep bedding over time. Your chicks will be raised here for the first three weeks.
- 10 to 15 cubic feet of fine pine shavings (two or three bags from Tractor Supply) for deep bedding in the brooder box. Start with 4 to 8 inches of bedding, then add whenever needed to keep up with the manure of your chicks.
- A 1-gallon waterer for the early brooder stage. After a couple of weeks, you'll need to shift to a 5-gallon waterer you'll use for the birds outside.
- Four 20-inch plastic tray feeders.
- Twenty-five 50-pound bags of starter feed. This is for the entire life cycle of your meat chickens, but it makes sense to order in bulk. I like the starter feed from New Country Organics.
- Grit placed in a small tray within the brooder.
- A gallon of Magic Water for your chicks' first watering. (That's 1 gallon of warm water, ½ cup of honey, ¼ cup of apple cider vinegar, and 4 cloves of minced garlic.)
- Two 150-watt clamp lamps.
- Two 150-watt red heat bulbs.
- Two large heat plates from Premier 1. Each plate accommodates fifty birds.
- Two Premier 1 poultry crates for transporting the birds out to grass, and then for collecting them at harvest.

Yes, there is a bit of an upfront investment there. But remember that you'll be able to reuse most of these supplies with future flocks of meat chickens.

Plan to move the chicks out of the brooder after about three weeks. At that point, you'll need some additional supplies to keep your young chickens safe and happy outside:

- Two 5-gallon poultry waterers.
- Two large automatic feeding systems. I like the King Feeders from Premier 1.
- One trough feeder. This looks like a really long open toolbox, and it's useful for making sure your birds have enough food at all times.
- Two food-grade buckets with lids. This is for carrying feed and filling up your different feeding stations.
- Netting to create pastures for the birds to move around in. I like the Shock-or-Not poultry net from Premier 1. (If you choose this option, make sure you also get the IntelliShock 60 Energizer.)

Introducing the MeatShaw

Just as we talked about with egg-layers, you'll need a system for managing and protecting your chickens while they're outside in the big, bad world. For meat chickens specifically, it really is best to get them out in the yard where they can walk, peck, and scratch in the grass or other vegetation. So, I don't recommend the Compost Corner setup for meat birds.

If you have twenty or fewer chickens, you can use the Chicken Tractor as your primary system. We covered that in Chapter 5, so I won't go into any more details here. If you're going to raise more than twenty birds, I recommend the MeatShaw, which is my own adaptation of the ChickShaw that is specifically designed for meat chickens.

There are several differences between raising meat chickens and egg-laying birds.

One of them is time. As we've already seen, your C-monsters will be ready for harvest in just eight weeks, while the dual-purpose egg-layers take up to six months or longer before they reach maturity and start to lay.

In terms of your chicken system, though, the biggest difference between egg-layers and meat chickens is that your C-monsters won't need a nesting place, since there won't be any eggs. In fact, because meat chickens are bigger and thicker, they generally stay on the ground. They don't need a perch to fly up to at night.

That's why the MeatShaw is so low to the ground. It's basically a roof on wheels, and it's designed primarily to offer your meat chickens protection from predators and the elements while they huddle together at night. It also

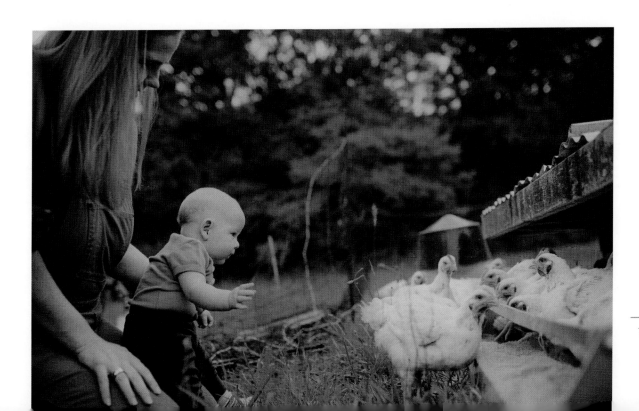

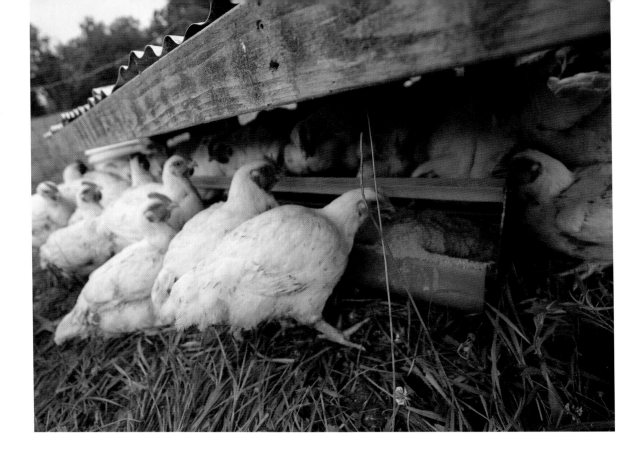

gives them a place to orient as their home, and lets them know where their food and water will be whenever they need it.

During the day, your C-monsters will mainly be out in the yard, pecking and scratching along like any other chickens within the confines of their netted pastures. But if they need some shade or if they get spooked by an aerial predator, the MeatShaw gives them a place to run for cover.

Speaking of pastures, you'll use the nets to create a pasture where the chickens can move around outside the MeatShaw if they feel like it—and, more importantly, where predators can't get in to bother the chickens. That's why I like the Shock-or-Not netting from Premier 1. The electric element is not intended to keep

your birds inside a specific area, but to keep predators out.

Now, as you might imagine, having a hundred chickens all huddled together under an 8 x 8-foot roof means a lot of chicken poop in a concentrated place—especially because chickens release half of their waste at night. That's why it's important to move the MeatShaw to a new spot every day.

To do this, just pull the whole apparatus forward the length of the MeatShaw. That includes moving your feeders and watering systems as well, since you want to keep everything close together for your birds. You should be able to move the MeatShaw three times within the space allowed by that Premier 1 netting. Then, on the fourth day, you'll need to move the net over to a new spot and start again in another three days.

The good news is that the chickens will mainly follow the MeatShaw when you're moving it or moving the nets. That's their home, and that's where the food is. So, they should stick close. If not, you can easily herd them into their new spot.

As always, you can find a detailed supply list and building plans for the MeatShaw at TheRootedLife.com/Resources.

The Glorious Guard Goose

I've mentioned a few times that chickens can be vulnerable to aerial predators, and that's something I know from experience. One year in particular, there was a hawk in our area who grabbed himself a chicken snack from my flock *every single day* for more than a week!

My first response was to pull all my birds under a Chicken Tractor so they were protected. (This was before I created the designs for my MeatShaw.) But as I kept reading, I came across another great idea from Joel Salatin: a Guard Goose.

After years of experience, I can confidently say that having a Guard Goose is one of the best and easiest ways to protect your chicken posse from both aerial and land predators. I say "best" because geese are large enough and scary enough to frighten away just about anything short of wolves. And I say "easiest" because geese get much of their food from foraging, and they do fine snacking on what you feed your chickens. Contrary to popular belief, geese do not need a body of water to thrive.

I recommend two tricks for making a Guard Goose work within your chicken system. First, raise your goose with the chicks. Meaning, you'll want to acquire a gosling from a hatchery and raise it as part of your chicken flock. That way it will think it's a chicken.

Second, get only one Guard Goose per flock. That's important because if you raise two or more geese together, they'll realize they're not chickens. They'll stick together and won't pay your chickens any mind—including not doing the work of protecting them from possible threats. The only problem here is that you typically have to order at least two waterfowl from any hatchery I know of. But, that means you'll have another goose to give away to a friend.

If you've got a Guard Goose on duty during the day, plus your electric net, you can nip 99 percent of your predator problems in the bud.

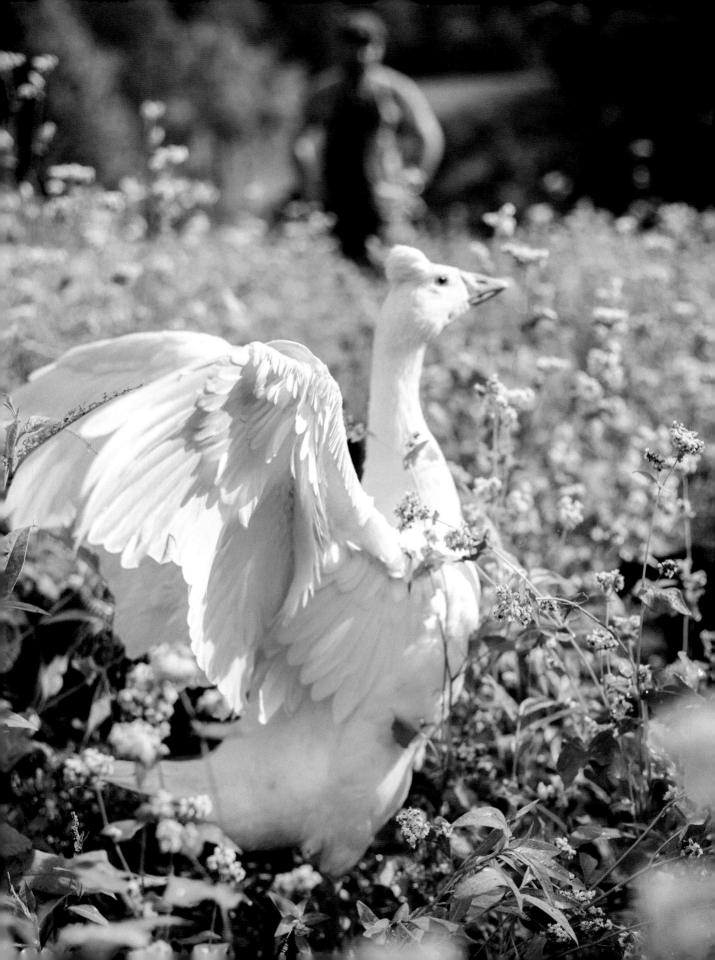

How to Make It Happen

By now I hope you can already taste that first bite of crispy fried chicken, just like your grandma used to make. Except yours will be even better, because it will be made with fresh, pasture-raised, healthy chicken you grew yourself.

The first thing you'll need to decide when you're ready to get started is how many chickens you want to raise. In general, raising a hundred chickens should give you plenty of meat to last a typical family over a typical year. But if your family can do well on one chicken a week, you may need only fifty chickens total.

Next is when to start. As I said earlier, it's best not to fight Mother Nature. The earliest you want to receive your C-monster chicks is three weeks before your last possible frost date. Ideally, you would start raising the chicks after that frost date. And certainly don't order chicks if you are less than eight weeks away from your first possible frost date in the fall.

In general, then, order your chicks in the spring and plan to harvest in the summer. (However, if you're living someplace really hot like Florida or Texas, you may want to try to raise your meat birds in the cooler seasons, such as spring or fall.)

Once you're ready to get started, here are the step-by-step instructions for growing your very own meat chickens:

Two weeks before the chicks arrive. Begin ordering your supplies. Also, it's good even at this point to have a plan for storing all your meat chickens once they're harvested. You should be able to fit about a hundred fully frozen birds in one good-size chest freezer.

Three days before the chicks arrive. Set up your brooder, making sure all the systems are in place and your lights and warmers are working well. Don't add any food or water just yet, but do put down a layer of 4 to 8 inches of pine shavings.

When the chicks arrive. Remember to turn on the brooder before you go to pick up the birds. I like having one heat lamp over the food and two heat plates for the chicks themselves. Also, mix up your Magic Water before you leave.

When you arrive with the chicks, put them in the brooder one at a time—dipping their beaks into the Magic Water before you set them on the pine shavings. Remember to keep count of how many chicks were actually shipped, and how many have survived.

Just as with egg-layers, it's a good idea to add a few handfuls of grass or other hand-torn greens to the brooder for the chicks to peck and enjoy.

The first two weeks. Make sure the chicks have access to food and water 24-7. No rationing here—you want the birds to grow quickly. Check on them at least twice a day and refill their food and water as needed.

During those checks, also make sure the chicks are warm. If you see them crowding each other or piling on top of each other around the heat sources, they may be too cold. Lower the heat lamp closer to the birds or add another heat source. If you see the chicks spreading out away from the heat sources, or if they're panting, they may be too hot. Lift the lamps away from the chicks or remove one of your heat sources.

Add a sprinkling of new pine shavings each day to keep the bedding dry and fresh. As always, if something starts to smell bad, add more bedding until the smell goes away. Keep adding grass or other greens each day.

Week three. Begin "hardening off" the chicks and getting them ready for the great outdoors by turning off their heat during the day for the first part of the week. Then, for the second part of the week, turn off their heat at night.

Week four. Plan to bring your C-monsters outside after three full weeks. It's best to make

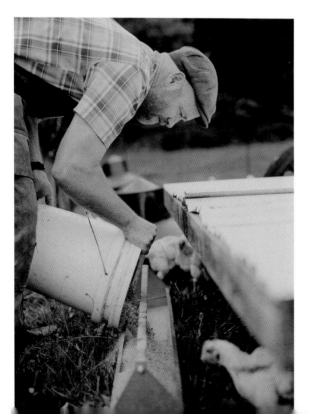

the transition during a dry afternoon. (If you need to wait until closer to four weeks because of rain or cold, that's okay.)

Set up the Shock-or-Not fencing around the MeatShaw wherever you plan to pasture the chickens first. We like to place our chickens in areas that need extra attention. That's because the manure produced by the C-monsters goes a long way toward boosting the land's fertility and restoring growth. To set up the net, I run it two post-lengths wide and five long. That narrow formation keeps the chickens relatively close to the coop and safe from aerial predators.

Collect the chicks in your poultry crates. You can fit fifty in one crate. Once you get inside the fence, dip your chicks' beaks into one of the waterers, then place them under the MeatShaw. This orients them to both the water and the MeatShaw. Do make sure you keep your feed and water close to the MeatShaw each day.

Finally, include a Guard Goose or install a scarecrow next to the fence. If you use a scarecrow, move it every three days with the chicks.

Four to eight weeks. Set your MeatShaw at one end of the fence and plan to move it inside the net every day. The MeatShaw will move three times in the space offered by one net, so you'll need to plan on moving the net every three days. (If you're feeling energetic, move your MeatShaw twice a day during the last week.) To move the net, simply pick it up, move your MeatShaw, feed, and water over to the next place, and set up everything as before.

Important: Don't be alarmed when the ground ends up being covered with manure. That's what chickens do! They may even kill the grass at first—but don't worry. After a short rest, that will become the greenest part of your yard or pasture.

Fill up the waterers and feeders in the morning when it's cool. Check on the water and feed each afternoon, refilling as needed. Usually, you won't have to refill in the afternoon until the last week or two. Up until that time, it's a good idea to shake your feeders to make sure food is coming down freely. (Sometimes it gets caught up in the automatic feeders.)

Six weeks. Start ordering and arranging your supplies for butchering. I also recommend you recruit some help if you can find it. Often you can pay people in chicken and a good meal. For example, we figure paying folks $16 an hour is fair, and we value our organic pasture-raised chicken at $6 a pound. So, if someone works eight hours, that's worth $128—or twenty-one pounds of chicken, which is roughly five birds. Other times folks are just eager to get the experience and won't even want compensation.

One or two days before butchering. Set up your butchering area and troubleshoot any problems.

Butchering day (eight weeks). You can go a few days past eight weeks if you need to, but no more than eight and a half. At that point, the C-monsters can grow too fast for their bones to keep up. Also, you risk not being able to fit them into your storage bags. Expect a 5-pound bird on average as you harvest. (You can weigh the birds alive and then reduce that number by 25 percent to get the freezer weight.)

We'll talk more about harvesting your meat chickens in Chapter 8. For now, just know it's not as bad as it sounds!

I said this in the chapter about egg-layers, but I want to say it again here because I think it's so important: Don't be afraid of chickens! If you've ever owned a dog and taken it out for a walk one or two times a day, you've already put in a similar amount of time and energy to what it will take to keep your birds going strong.

Raising chickens for meat is not only a fantastic way to add nutrient-rich meat to your table each and every week, it's also a great way to be part of the story of feeding your family. You get in there and sustain the lives of your feathered friends as a means of sustaining the lives of your loved ones.

In short, whether for eggs or meat, raising chickens is a great way to pursue the rooted life.

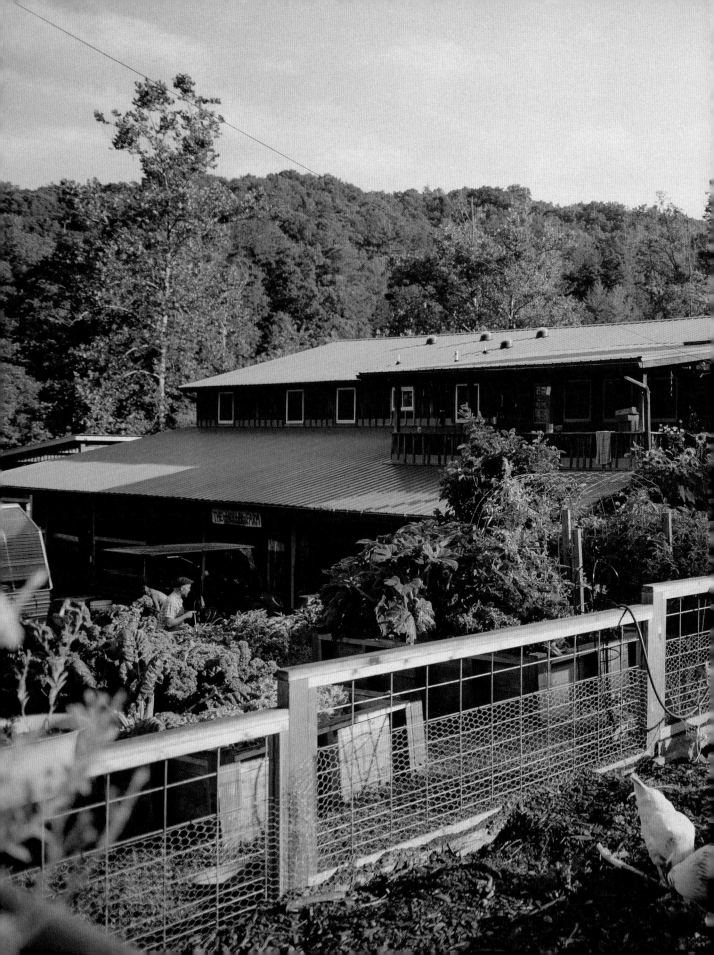

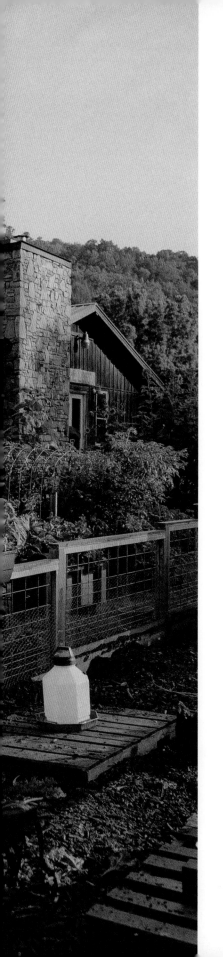

CHAPTER 7

Sweet Synergy: Gardening with Chickens

It was late at night. I was in bed, the Beautiful One beside me reading a book. I was just slipping into that sweet spot between consciousness and sleeping bliss when I felt it: Rebekah poked me. That happens to be a pet peeve of mine, so I ignored it and continued my journey toward Dreamland.

"Justin." She poked me again.

I half opened one eye and said the only thing I could think of that wouldn't be rude. "Yes?" Actually, I might have put a little pepper into those three letters. Maybe an exclamation point. "Yes?!"

"Did you put up the chickens?" By the tone of her voice I could tell she already knew the answer. So did I.

"No."

"Well, are you gonna?"

That's when I said it—a bitter burst of bile that surprised even me. "Sometimes I just wish they'd *die*!"

Did I really mean what I said? In that moment, yes. A hundred percent. This was about ten years into our homestead journey, which meant I'd already put up those blasted chickens nearly 4,000 times. On top of that, I'd recently been diagnosed with chronic Lyme disease, which meant my physical energy was drained and my mental capacity kaput. I felt tired, frustrated, and defeated. I just wanted to go to sleep.

Of course, I didn't go to sleep. Of course, I did stumble my way downstairs and put the chickens up. And of course I grumbled about it the whole way there and back.

But I also made a decision. Something had to change. There had to be a better way to run things—a more efficient way to manage all the different elements of our homestead, especially given the recent reduction in my energy levels. If I could find that better way, great. Otherwise, I decided, I was done. I would throw in the towel and find something else to do with my life.

Permaculture Power

I'll spare you the long, drawn-out story—but I did find what I was looking for. Specifically, I found a concept called Permaculture that literally changed the way I managed everything on our homestead. I even flew from North Carolina to Australia to meet and learn from Geoff Lawton, one of the leaders of the modern Permaculture movement.

What is Permaculture? At the core, it's a design concept that seeks to make connections between the different elements within an environment (such as your homestead). Permaculture isn't a gardening technique, nor is it a system for raising chickens. Instead, Permaculture is like the toolbox in which gardening and chickens sit. It's the design behind those systems that maximizes efficiency, health, and productivity.

Long story short, implementing the Permaculture concepts I picked up instantly made my farm more productive with less effort. Not just mine, either. I've helped thousands of people benefit from those same principles through our website (AbundancePlus.com) and our YouTube videos. That's good news for you as well. I've flown to Australia, read all the books, and implemented the concepts myself with blood, sweat, and tears—all so you can learn the most important principles in these pages without making the same mistakes.

Actually, you've already been learning about those principles within these pages. Remember "Start right outside your front door"? That's a core element of Permaculture. Geoff taught me to think of all the different pieces of my homestead as "elements"— Container Gardens, Bulletproof Gardens, Crop Gardens, egg chickens, meat chickens, cows, pigs, ducks, greenhouses, fruit trees, woods, and

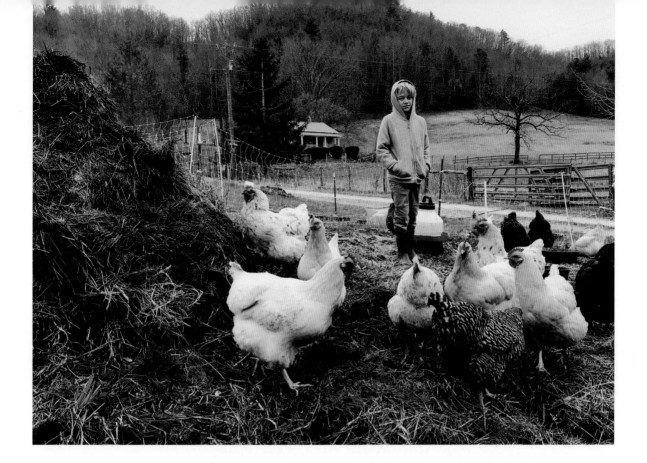

so on. Everything within my homestead is an element.

Geoff encouraged me to determine which elements I visited most during a typical day and a typical week. (That was easy: my chickens!) Then he suggested I maximize efficiency by placing the elements I visited most frequently closest to my front door.

Another important principle in Permaculture is to combine elements that are mutually beneficial. Like the Guard Goose, for example. Chickens need protection from predators, and geese need food and social interaction. Well, if you put a single goose in with the chickens, you are meeting both of those needs with minimum effort and maximum efficiency.

I encourage you to take a moment to think through the different elements within your own home or yard. Make a list of everything there—animals, gardens, container plants, trees, a creek if you have one, and so on. Then evaluate each of those elements by asking two questions: (1) What does it need?, and (2) What does it provide?

Once you've got everything on paper, you might be surprised how many needs within those elements can be directly met by what another element provides. For example, if you have a field with lots of weeds or scrub or other unwanted vegetation, that field needs to be cleaned out regularly. Well, if you've got some devil's eyes (goats), they need food. Quite a lot of food. Boom! Put the goats in the field, and you've got Permaculture—each element meeting the needs of the other.

This brings us to the third Permaculture principle I want to highlight briefly: turning problems into solutions. Selah, the farm manager at Geoff Lawton's Zaytuna Farm in Australia, told us, "The core of the problem is the seed for a solution." I love that idea! More importantly, it works.

Remember in Chapter 3 when I talked about harvesting your bugs? That's a great example of this principle. If there are bugs eating up your gardens, that's a problem.

If left unmanaged, they will cause a lot of damage to your crops. But you can turn that problem into a solution by harvesting those bugs and throwing them to your chickens as feed. (Actually, that's turning a problem into delicious chicken and eggs!)

That's only a very quick introduction to the ideas and principles behind the Permaculture movement. If you want to learn more, you can find several books and websites to explore on our Resources page at the back of this book (page 191).

Chickens and Gardens

If you're wondering why I've gone down the Permaculture rabbit trail in a chapter about gardening with chickens, the answer is it's not a rabbit trail at all. I can't think of a better example of Permaculture principles at work than the sweet synergy between gardens and chickens.

As we've seen, gardens and chickens can be important elements not only for farms and homesteads, but for any family that has a little

extra space and a little extra time to invest in growing their own food. Not only that, both of those elements—gardens and chickens—have things they need and things they provide.

What I want to show you over the rest of this chapter is how remarkably well gardens and chickens work together to provide for each other's needs—and how well they can maximize your efforts to cultivate health and wellness for your family.

Before the Growing Season

There are two main ways chickens can provide for the needs of your gardens before the growing season: by creating compost and by

preparing those garden beds for planting. Let's start with compost.

If you have a stationary chicken coop

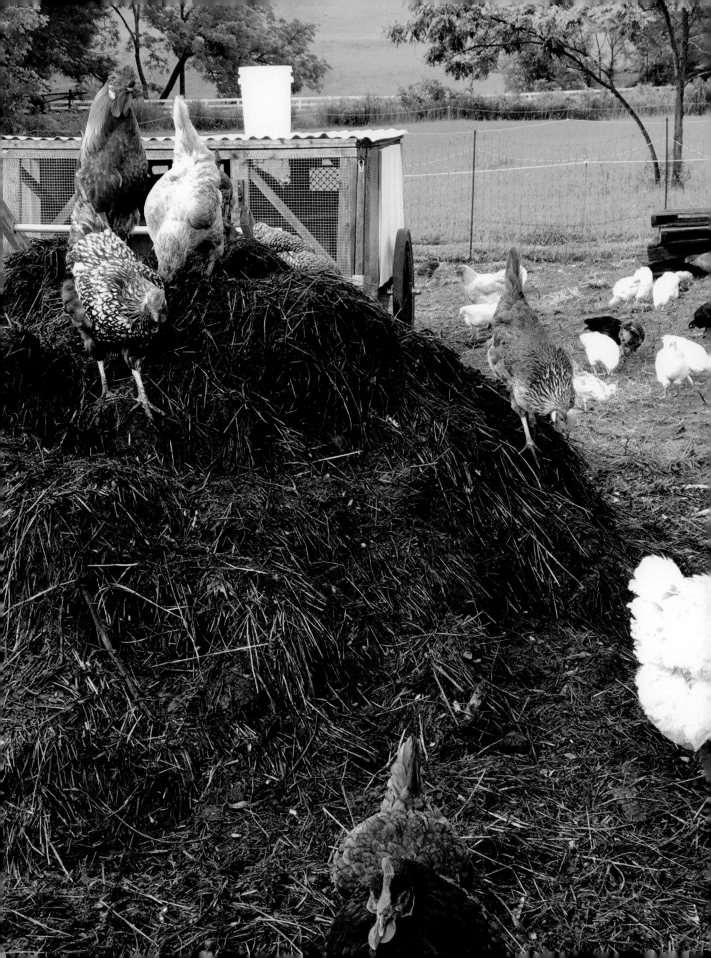

or house—and especially if you're using something like the Compost Corner I described in Chapter 5—then your chickens have worked for months throughout the fall, winter, and early spring to create something lovely for your gardens: compost. Sometimes I call it "black gold," because it's that valuable for supercharging the growing power of your gardens.

Here's how it works: When your chickens poop in a stationary pen, the waste falls on the deep bedding under their nests or in the chicken run. Then the chickens do what they do, scratching all day long, and eventually that manure (which happens to be high in nitrogen) gets mixed into the bedding. Over time, the carbon in that bedding gets broken down by the nitrogen and the surrounding air, which produces compost. After about six months, you'll be able to harvest a good batch of compost, which can be used directly on your gardens or raised beds.

Here's how to harvest the compost once you're ready to prepare your gardens for spring planting:

- Use a hard rake to pull away the surface of the deep bedding until you see black (fresh-smelling) compost below. If there's no black soil underneath, you don't have compost yet. You'll get compost faster when your deep bedding sits directly on the soil.
- Dig out the compost using a shovel, but try not to dig into the actual soil below.
- Place a sifter on top of a wheelbarrow or garden cart, and then shovel your compost into that. For a homemade sifter, I attached a ½-inch hardware cloth to a 30 x 30-inch frame that easily rests on my wheelbarrow. Works great.
- Now, take your shovel and just scrape the compost back and forth across the mesh until all the fine compost has fallen through and all the larger unbroken pieces—wood chips, soil chunks, rocks, or whatever—stay in the sifter. Throw the larger stuff back and wheelbarrow your fresh compost wherever it needs to go.

If you don't have a stationary chicken house or a Compost Corner, that's okay. You can still get compost by placing a layer of deep bedding (4 to 8 inches) underneath a mobile coop such as the Chicken Tractor. Leave that mobile coop on top of the deep bedding for a couple of weeks or more, then pull it off. You'll be left with a combination of bedding and manure. All you need to do from that point on is stir that pile a few times, then let it sit. Nature will do the work of transforming it into compost.

The second way chickens can provide for your gardens before the growing season is by preparing those gardens and beds for planting. This happens when you allow the chickens to "graze" on top of those gardens—by using a mobile coop like the Chicken Tractor or ChickShaw and/or setting up temporary nets to create pastures for your chickens.

One thing that happens when you let chickens into garden beds is that they "till" the ground by scratching and pecking constantly, which is just what chickens do. You can encourage this natural behavior by feeding your chickens directly on the ground. Better still, as they go about this important work, they also drop packets of manure into the garden, fertilizing the soil.

Chickens also debug the soil by gobbling up ticks, ants, crickets, fly larvae, mosquito larvae, or any other bugs that happen to be in the neighborhood. In a single day, a little posse of chickens can break pest cycles that have hampered your gardens for years!

Notice it's not just the gardens that benefit from this synergy. Your chickens will get fresh air, fresh greens, and fresh bugs in return for their hard work. (You'll benefit as well, because chickens who have access to sunlight and fresh greens will lay omega-rich eggs packed full of vitamins.)

Also, after the chickens have prepped a garden area, you can build a Bulletproof Garden or Crop Garden there. (See my Instant Chicken Garden on page 124 for instructions.)

During the Growing Season

Before the growing season, it's primarily the chickens who "feed" the gardens by providing compost and prepping the grounds. Once seeds are planted, however, those roles reverse. During the growing seasons, it's the gardens that feed the chickens.

The first way this happens is through weeds. As I've already mentioned, one of the chores you'll need to keep track of during the growing season is weeding your gardens. Container Gardens, Bulletproof Gardens, Crop Gardens—all of them grow weeds, although you can minimize that growth by using a silage tarp for your larger plots or mulch for smaller ones.

So, once a week—maybe twice during

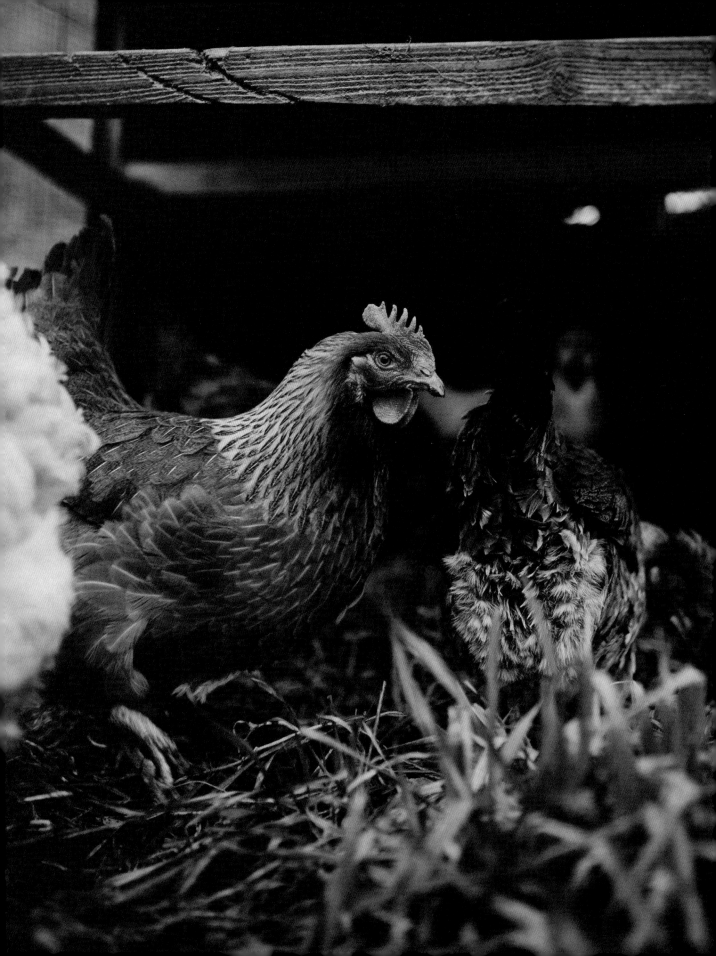

peak growth—you'll need to go through your gardens and pull any weeds. But don't toss them into the garbage can! Don't even throw them out in the woods to decompose. Instead, toss them to your chickens so they can have fresh greens to eat. Whatever they don't eat they'll shred into compost.

See how powerful Permaculture can be? Weeds are a problem, but you can turn them into a solution by using them as chicken food.

Incidentally, this is another reason why it's good to place your gardens and chickens physically close together whenever possible.

That way you can pull up a few weeds, turn around, and literally just toss them over the fence into your chicken run. No need to walk back and forth.

The other way your gardens will feed your chickens is through food scraps. Once you start harvesting produce, obviously your family will eat it—or most of it, anyway. There's always something left over. Stalks, inedible leaves, portions that go bad or sit in the fridge for too long. Once again, don't throw those away. Instead, contribute to the circle of life by tossing those scraps to your feathered friends.

After the Growing Season

Once you've finished harvesting in a specific garden or raised bed, it's time to move your chicken posse back in and let them run free once more. Those chickens will do a fantastic job of cleaning up any leftover vegetation—weeds, the remains of your crops, vines, and so on. The chickens will also keep up their usual work of debugging, tilling, fertilizing, and more.

Usually it takes only a couple of days for the chickens to clean things out—two weeks, max. Then you can move them out. If the chickens are cleaning out a Bulletproof Garden, I recommend you add 6 to 8 inches of mulch after they finish. If they have finished working on a Crop Garden, just reshape the beds, put down an inch or two of compost, and then cover with a silage tarp until it's time to plant again.

Once again, this is a great system for both the gardens and the chickens. Each element is both giving and receiving, which gives each element a better chance of thriving.

Example: The Instant Chicken Garden

I mentioned earlier in the book how the COVID-19 pandemic created a huge wave of people who became interested in growing their own food. What I haven't mentioned is how Rebekah and I tried to help.

During those early months in 2020, we kept getting requests from people to teach them about homesteading, gardening, and raising chickens. Many of these folks were new to our website and our YouTube channel. Most of them wanted to start a garden and start raising chickens ASAP—they were seriously ready for some food security—but they didn't have much land and didn't really know the basics.

As I was thinking about how to help these folks, I considered that Rebekah and I had already planted several fast-growing, cold-hardy crops such as spinach, lettuce, and kale. Those crops would be ready for harvest in just sixty days. Two months! I realized I could teach people how to set up a high-efficiency food-growing system that doesn't take up much space, yields lots of veggies quickly, *and* produces eggs! I called it the Instant Chicken Garden, and it was a huge success.

You should consider this chicken-garden combo if you:

- Have a little space and want to combine your gardens with three or four chickens.
- Want a garden right away.
- Want to maximize the amount of food you can grow in a small space.
- Have access to grass clippings, organic straw, leaves, or wood chips.
- Can afford the $350 start-up costs for my DIY Chicken Tractor.

The basic idea for the Instant Chicken Garden is to use chickens as the primary tool for quickly and efficiently preparing a section of your yard to become a Bulletproof Garden. As always, you'll need to find a relatively flat, sunny space for the garden. And ideally you'll want that space to be as close to your front door as possible so that you can maintain the garden easily. (In an ideal world, you'd plant your Instant Chicken Garden right next to your Compost Corner or other chicken coop, and both would be right next to your house.)

To make this happen, you'll need the materials for the Bulletproof Garden I listed in Chapter 3. You'll also need to construct a DIY Chicken Tractor. (You can find that supply list and instructions at TheRootedLife.com/Resources.) Finally, you'll need three to five dual-purpose chickens to both work the ground and eventually lay some eggs.

Once you've got all the supplies, here are the basic steps for using chickens to create a quick, vibrant garden right outside your front door.

Step 1. Find a relatively flat area in the part of your yard that gets the most sun. You'll need at least 3 x 8 feet to make room for your Chicken Tractor and leave space for you to move around. If you're planning on more than one garden area, leave 12 to 18 inches for a path between beds. Nine garden beds would be the perfect amount because you could start with Garden #1, plant whatever crops you choose (including things like pumpkins that take 120 days to mature), and move the tractor to a new bed every two weeks. By the time you're done with the ninth bed, you will have harvested from Garden #1, which means you can bring the chickens back to clean it up.

Step 2. Set up your Chicken Tractor on your future garden spot with three or four adult laying chickens. Feed them every day on the ground to encourage tilling.

Now, this is the important point: *Don't move the Chicken Tractor.* Keep it on that same bed for two weeks. Normally this would be a bad idea because the chickens would tear up the sod and kill the grass—that's why I encourage people to build mobile chicken coops that can be moved to a new spot every day.

For the Instant Chicken Garden, however, you *want* the chickens to tear through that sod. You want the grass to be killed (and probably eaten as well, which is great for the eggs your chickens will lay).

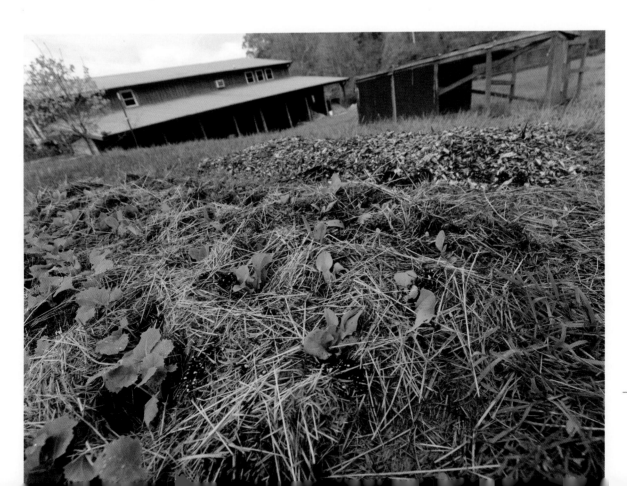

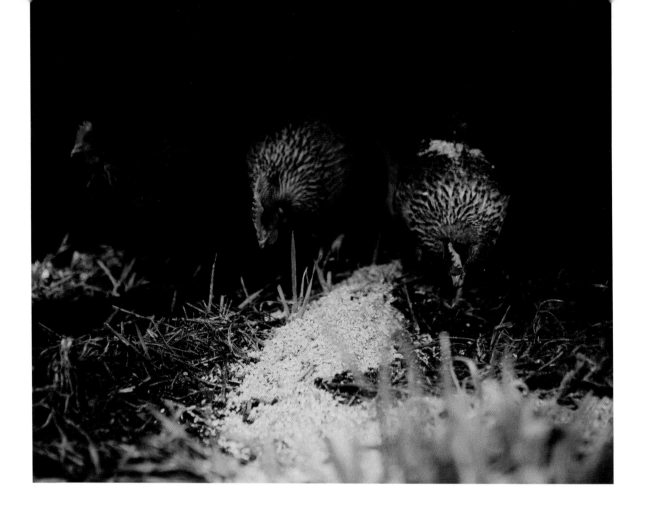

That way the ground will be fully tilled and prepared by the time you are ready to plant your crops in two weeks.

Step 3. After two weeks, go ahead and move your Chicken Tractor away from the garden. (Remember, you can move it just 18 inches away to start prepping a second bed, then a third, and so on.) You'll find a rectangular plot of ground with little or no grass and lots of chicken droppings. That's great! It's a wonderful start for a fertile growing environment.

The first thing you need to do is rake the manure around so that it's spread evenly over your garden bed. Then sprinkle a few food scraps on the ground as worm food. If your soil requires any amendments, add them here.

Step 4. Lay down at least 3 inches of compost spread over your 3 x 8-foot garden bed. (Again, if you've got a Compost Corner with deep bedding, you should be able to provide most or all of the compost you'll need for these gardens.)

Step 5. Lay down a 3 x 8-foot piece of weed paper on top of the compost, then soak it.

Step 6. Put 4 inches of grass clippings or other mulch on top of the paper and wet again.

Step 7. If you're growing your own plant starts from seeds, begin hardening them off at around three weeks.

Step 8. Two weeks after you have moved out the Chicken Tractor and put down your compost and mulch, your beds should be ready for planting. Transplant the starts into the garden—remember to space out each crop based on its needs—and water a full inch immediately afterward to help the plants handle the stress of their move. At this point, you can just walk away if you want to. But if you want to weed and add an inch of water each week it doesn't rain, that will only help things grow.

Step 9. Harvest the bounty! Remember that different plants take different amounts of time to mature, and some plants (such as cabbages, lettuces, and kale) can be harvested for several weeks by removing only the outer layers every few days.

Step 10. Once the harvest is finished, bring your chickens back in to glean any remaining produce and eat up any weeds, vines, or other leftover greens. And of course, if you're working with mature chickens, you can be harvesting eggs this whole time. That's the beauty of the Instant Chicken Garden—fresh produce and fresh eggs in a ridiculously quick amount of time.

Here's something else to think about: If you have a lot of chickens, you can scale up this idea by using a ChickShaw (or even multiple ChickShaws) to prepare a Crop Garden. The principle would be the same as for the Instant Chicken Garden, just bigger. In my experience, twenty-four chickens can prep a brand-new 24 x 50-foot garden bed in four to six weeks. The same chickens can prep an existing garden in just a few days.

———

So there you have it: Chickens and gardens go together like bacon and eggs. Like peanut butter and chocolate. Like—well, you get the idea. Trust me, I've been a witness to this synergy for more than a decade now, and it's far and away one of the most powerful steps you can take in your journey toward the rooted life.

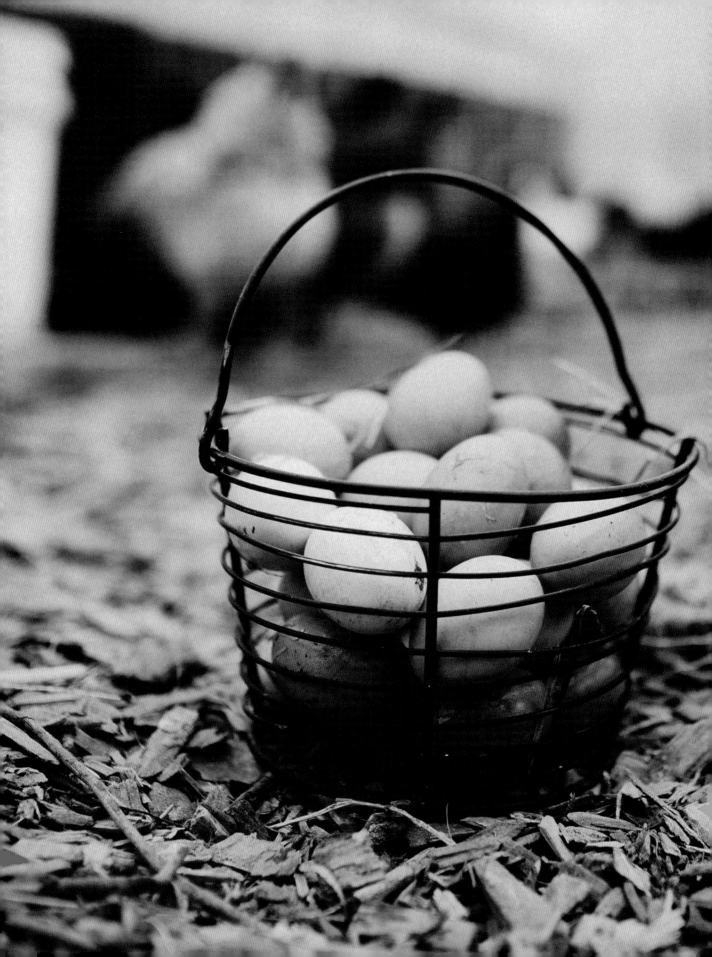

CHAPTER 8

The Joy of the Harvest

I was walking through the bottom level of our house barn when I looked over at the chicken stall and saw it—saw *them*. I started to take another step closer to make sure I was really seeing what I was seeing, but there wasn't much doubt. I was sure. I ran out of the barn and up the stairs toward our living room.

"Rebekah!" I was already calling her name when I burst through the door. She was folding clothes or something, as if it was a normal day. She had no idea what was coming.

"Rebekah, we've got eggs!"

Let me rewind a little bit. After the fiasco with our first chickens—you remember Uno, Dos, Tres, and Quatro, right?—we eventually decided to try again with some new chicks. Thankfully, this time we had our act together. We got each of our birds oriented correctly in that basement stall, and we had a good system going for feeding and caring for them.

We placed our order for those chicks in the spring, and we knew it would take about six months before they started laying eggs. So we waited. And waited. And kept waiting a little more. Finally, it was fall. The time had come. The stall was filled with full-size chickens, and we knew they should start laying those eggs any moment now. We were excited!

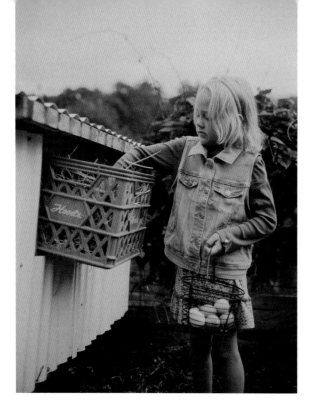

Well, any moment now became any day now. And any day now became any week now. But there was nothing. No eggs. Rebekah and I kept going about our chores, and every day we'd stop by the stall and check to see if the first egg had been laid. Sometimes several times a day. Still nothing. Still no eggs.

Eventually we stopped checking. At least I did. Honestly, I somehow got into the mindset that it was never going to happen. We must have bought some dud chickens. I gave up.

Then the day came when I walked into that stall and just happened to glance over at the chickens—and there they were. Not just a first egg, but eggs. Close to a dozen! If you've never raised chickens, the first eggs a hen lays are always tiny. So, these were itty-bitty eggs, but I didn't care! I ran up the stairs to find my wife.

Once I told her the good news, Rebekah shouted for joy right along with me. Then, always the practical thinker, she asked, "Aren't you going to bring them up?" Woops. In my excitement I'd left them all down in the stall. That's how overjoyed I was.

Even today when people tell me about harvesting their first eggs, I'm taken back to that moment, and I feel those emotions all over again—because it worked! Because six months of effort and expense had finally paid off.

I did go back down and get those eggs, and our family had breakfast for dinner that night to celebrate. It was glorious.

You're going to have lots of those moments as you pursue the rooted life. Lots of those meals and celebrations. Think of how amazing it will feel when you make that first salad where you grew every ingredient. Think of your counter stacked with squashes and your fridge packed with fresh veggies. Think of cooking with your own fresh herbs. Oh, and think of that first crispy bite of fried chicken!

Now think of how you'll feel when you look over your finances and see that grocery bill going down. Then down some more. You're eating a much higher quality of food and you're paying much less for the privilege. Maybe you'll even get to the point where you can sell your extra food and make a profit!

Those are the goals and moments I want you to keep at the front of your mind as you keep flipping these pages. Because they really can happen. They really *will* happen— including the joy of the harvest.

Knowing When It's Time to Harvest

Gardening or growing any kind of food is always a waiting game. That was true all the way back in elementary school when you planted your first bean seed in that little cup—remember how excited you were to see that tiny green shoot poke its way up through the soil, and how long it took?—and it's still true today.

The question many people have is: How do I know when the waiting is over? How can I tell when what I've grown is ready for harvest?

The technical answer is that you can check the instructions on the packaging of your seeds or plant starts to determine how long it takes each plant to reach maturity. For example, spinach will go from a seed to ready to eat in about forty-five days. But remember, those instructions are more guidelines than hard-and-fast rules. There's always going to be some fluctuation.

The best way to determine when it's time to harvest your food is to use your eyes. Meaning, when something looks good enough to eat, it's ready for harvest. When those lettuce leaves are comparable to what you typically buy in the store, it's time to harvest. The same is true when your pumpkins, tomatoes, and peppers have lost all their green and are fully colored.

Trust your eyes!

Another question I hear on this topic is how often to check different crops to determine whether they are ready for harvest. Should you go out there and poke through your plants every day to see whether something looks good enough to eat? Maybe multiple times a day if you're getting close? No. The point of growing your own food is to add convenience and reduce stress, not the other way around.

If you've got a Container Garden or a Bulletproof Garden, hopefully you've taken my advice and set that up pretty close to your front door. So if you're coming home and have a minute, sure, take a quick look and see if anything is ready for harvest. Checking any more than once a day is just wasting time.

For the sake of efficiency, the best option is to check over your plants once or twice a week.

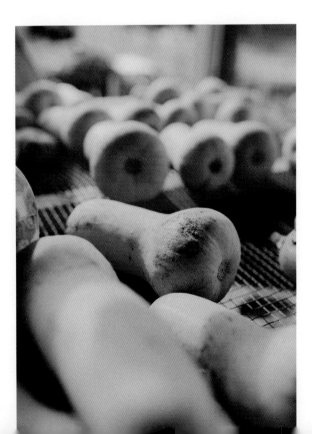

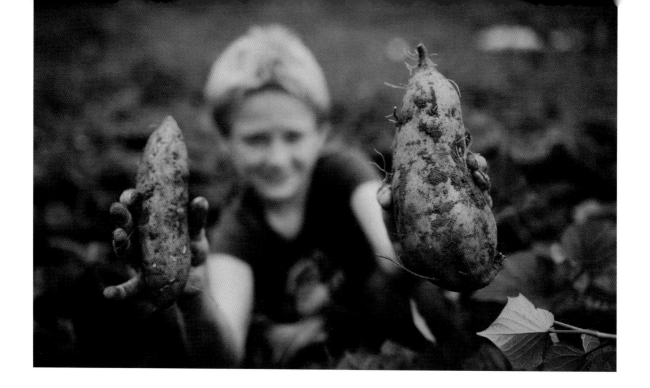

Remember, you're already going to be watering and weeding once a week. As the growing season progresses and you get close to harvest-time, just add a harvest check to those regular chores and you'll be good to go.

One final reminder: If you plant your gardens after the last possible frost date for your climate zone, you will maximize your growing season, which will maximize your harvest. Play your cards right and you can even get multiple harvests within a single growing season.

Tips and Tricks for the Harvest

You put in the work on the front end by filling containers, spreading compost, and shaping beds. You planted your seeds or starts with great anticipation and great hope. You've spent the past several weeks cultivating and maintaining your crops by keeping everything weeded and watered—and now your eyes are telling you it's time to reap your reward.

Time to harvest! This is what you've been waiting for, and this is the moment that makes all your work worthwhile. Enjoy it.

In my experience, there are two basic approaches when it comes to harvesting your homegrown food. The first is what I call an "as you need it" style of harvesting, which works best with Container Gardens and Bulletproof Gardens. This method basically treats your gardens as an extension of your pantry or refrigerator.

Need some tomatoes for your patented spaghetti sauce? Walk out to your garden and grab a couple. (It's easy because you planted your garden right outside your front door.) Need a little more peppermint for your tea? Just break off a sprig or two from the container on your windowsill. It's easy as can be. Or, if you're the kind of person who likes to plan ahead, harvest a few days' worth of produce—whatever you plan to eat or use in recipes during that time span. Then, when you've gone through that, go out and harvest a little more.

Let me tell you, this type of harvesting beats the pants off of running out to the grocery store!

The other way to approach a harvest is simply to make it another chore on your homestead and tackle it once a week—or maybe twice a week if you've got lots of food ready to go. I call this the "all at once" style of harvesting, and it's necessary if you've got Crop Gardens. For this method, you go through each of your gardens and gather everything that's ready to be harvested (whether you're ready to use it or not). This approach is more efficient in the long run, but it will require a good chunk of work on the day you do your harvesting. It will also require places and methods to store or preserve what you harvest (more on that below).

Rebekah and I usually take this once-a-week approach to harvesting, although it's certainly nice to be able to access a lot of great food if there's something specific we need. Just last night, for example, our family was cooking hamburgers when we realized we had no lettuce. We sent one of our little ones out with a strainer to fill with lettuce leaves, washed what she brought in, and boom—it was burger time.

That's the joy of the harvest!

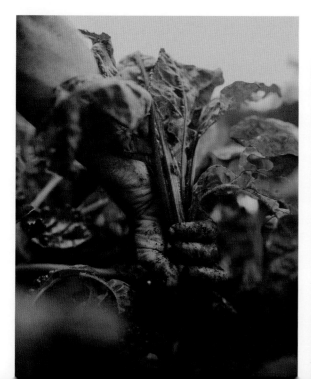
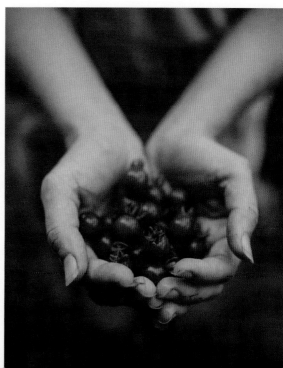

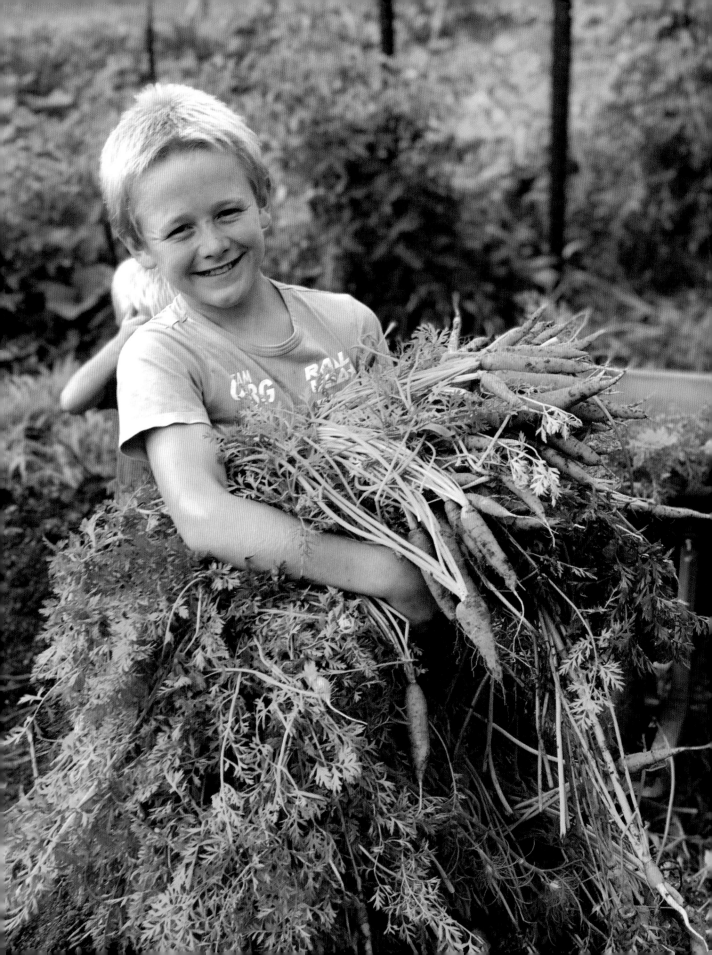

What You'll Need

The good news is you don't need much in terms of supplies to bring off a successful harvest. The biggest thing you'll need is a container (or several containers, depending on the size of the harvest) to gather what you pick. This can be anything from a canvas bag or a little plastic tub all the way up to a wheelbarrow.

Then, if the harvest is big enough, you will need some containers or storage options to keep your produce fresh until you're ready to use it. For example, Rebekah and I often harvest a lot of squash, which is a food that keeps really well even at room temperature. You can leave an acorn squash or a butternut squash just sitting on your counter for up to six months, and it will still be good when you're ready to eat it. We built some shelves in our storage area that are specifically designed to keep our squash for long periods of time.

If you're harvesting from a Container Garden or a Bulletproof Garden, you will likely be fine with your refrigerator and whatever you currently use as a pantry. If you're harvesting a Crop Garden, you'll need to look into more-involved options for storing your produce,

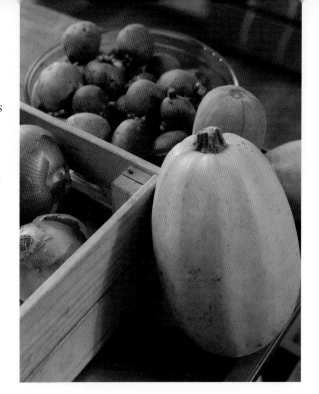

which can include anything from canning to freezing and beyond.

One other tool I recommend you have for harvesttime is a good sharp knife. A knife is important because you want to avoid yanking your food away from stems or stalks, which can damage the growing portions of your plants. Instead, use your knife to cut things free quickly and cleanly. You can also pinch off or twist fruits such as tomatoes, cucumbers, apples, and so on.

Harvesting Specific Crops

Some common plants and produce require a little extra know-how come harvesttime, so let's walk through the main examples together.

Leafy greens. The great thing about leafy greens is that you can harvest one plant for weeks at a time. If you have a nice head of lettuce ready to harvest, for example, you can peel off or cut away those outer leaves and throw them in your salad. If you keep the central leaves in place, they will keep growing—which means you can come back in a couple of days and harvest some more lettuce from that same plant.

This works for lettuce, kale, spinach, Swiss chard, and collards. Eventually the plant will stop producing, and that's when you can use your knife to cut away the whole head or batch.

Root crops. These are crops that grow in the ground, which means you'll need to dig up one or two to do a harvest check and eventually to harvest. Many times you can wiggle the stalks back and forth a little bit to loosen things up and pull the crop partly out of the ground. If it's not ready, gently ease it back down into the soil.

Examples of these crops are carrots, beets, turnips, onions, ginger, and radishes.

Potatoes and sweet potatoes. These are also root crops, but they function a little differently. First, you can get a good sense of when your potato crop is ready to harvest by watching the vine growing above the ground. When that vine dries up and dies, your potatoes are ready.

At that point, you'll need a spade or potato fork to dig the tubers out of the ground. It's always a good idea to dig when your soil is relatively dry because the potatoes will come up more easily. Also, do your best not to scrape or cut the tubers during the process, because damaged produce has a much greater tendency to rot in storage.

Harvesting Eggs and Chickens

Harvesting Eggs

Chickens lay their eggs primarily in the morning. Sometimes you might see a new egg early in the afternoon, but that's rare. So, the easiest way to harvest your eggs is to gather them when you put the chickens up to rest. The timing here is important because it's good to harvest the eggs before the colder temperatures at night (in case of freezing), and it is possible for chickens to get bored before they go to bed and start pecking at any eggs lying around.

Gathering the eggs is super simple.

You'll walk into the coop or chicken house—wherever the chickens sleep at night—and you'll see the eggs just lying in the nesting places. All you need to do is scoop them up and put them in a basket or other storage container.

Here's another thing many people don't know about fresh eggs: They can last up to six or eight weeks sitting on your counter. Unrefrigerated. (Just don't wash them.) That's because all chicken eggs come out with a natural film that seals and protects them—I

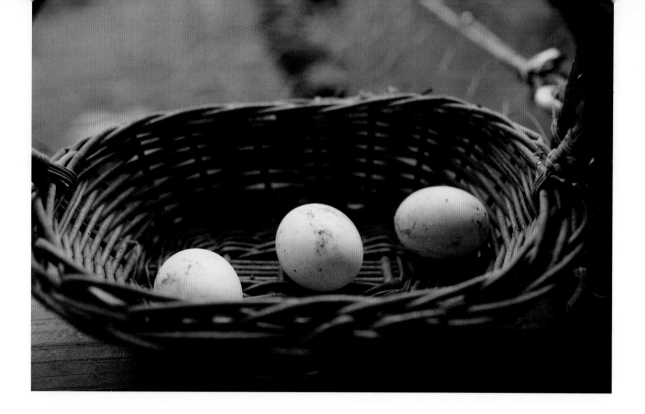

call it God's Goop. If you were to see a chicken actually laying, the egg would appear wet or slick. It dries pretty quickly, so you won't see it most of the time. But it still does its work of protecting the egg from bacteria and keeping it fresh for weeks at a time.

Now, there are times when eggs get dirty before you can grab them—maybe a little poopy or muddy. In that case, you do want to wash off the egg. That means you'll wash off God's Goop as well, so you'll need to put that egg in the refrigerator, where it will still be fresh and usable for a week or two, just like eggs you buy at the store.

One question I often get about harvesting eggs is how to tell whether an egg is rotten. First, if the egg has a bad smell to it before you crack it, then it's rotten. Get rid of it. If you have suspicions about an egg but you can't

quite tell, drop it into a cup of water. If the egg floats, it's rotten.

One more tip: When you do crack an egg, save the shell. Crush it up and feed it back to your chickens. Just toss it into their pasture or chicken run or wherever you keep them. Those crushed shells are a calcium source, and your chickens can munch on them if they need a little extra calcium boost—which happens when they're laying often. (Note: It's important to crush the shells so your chickens don't start pecking at whole eggs looking for a snack.)

Harvesting Meat Chickens

I'll just come out and say it: Nobody likes butchering chickens. I understand that. It's messy work, and the first few times it can make you a little queasy. That's one of the reasons why raising chickens for meat isn't a good option for everyone.

The good news for those who do decide to raise their own meat chickens is that butchering isn't really that bad once you get used to it. It's not rocket science, that's for sure! Anyone can learn to do it. Best of all, when you raise meat chickens, you typically have to worry about butchering only once a year.

Here are the basic steps for humanely butchering a chicken:

- Twelve hours before you harvest your chickens, stop feeding them so their crops will be empty. (If you're not going to butcher all your birds, just herd the ones to be harvested into a separate pen or pasture.)

- When the time has come, place the chicken in a restraining cone to prevent any slipping, then quickly slice the bird's neck as close as you can get toward the cheek bone. Then slice the other side. Bend the bird's head to encourage bleeding. (If you don't see much blood, you probably need to cut again.) It should take about three minutes for all the blood to drain.

- Drop the chicken into a large bucket of scalding water and gently move it with tongs or a poker. (Not boiling water— about 145°F is best.) After thirty to sixty seconds, move the chicken to a bucket of cold water.

- Now it's time to pluck the feathers. You can do this by hand, but a machine is about ten times faster. If you plan to harvest a lot of birds, I recommend a machine. (Or a bunch of volunteers!)

- Put the bird on its back and make a horizontal slit just up from the tailbone and vent. Now, pull open the carcass with your fingers and remove the excess appendages, organs, and entrails. This will typically include the bird's head, legs, and feet, plus everything on the inside you don't intend to eat. The guts will still be attached to the vent, but now that they are outside of the body, you should be able to slice down the left and right side of the vent, then below the vent, to completely remove the vent and guts without piercing the intestines.

- At this point you'll probably recognize the chicken as pretty close to what you buy from the store. Rinse everything with water, and then place in a cooler for packaging. You can freeze the entire chicken whole, or you can cut it into pieces.

That doesn't sound so bad, does it? If you're ready to harvest your own meat chickens, we've got supply lists, step-by-step instructions, and even a video walk-through at TheRootedLife .com/Resources.

Preserving the Harvest

Rebekah and I have served as foster parents many times over the years, and especially early on in our marriage. One of the things that was special about those experiences was introducing kids who "don't like vegetables" to how healthy, organic food is supposed to taste.

For example, we had one young lady who used to spend weekends at our home. She probably had never eaten a vegetable before she came to us. But I can still see her in my mind's eye standing out there in our garden and munching away on a raw ear of corn. No butter. No salt. Not even cooked. She just loved that raw sweet corn because it was so fresh and so packed with flavor. I still smile when I think of those moments. They were a joy to watch.

I love seeing my own chiddlers doing the same thing. Let me tell you: When our berry patches are producing fruit, those kids get after it! They can't get enough of those fresh strawberries, blueberries, and blackberries. There have been days when we had to literally

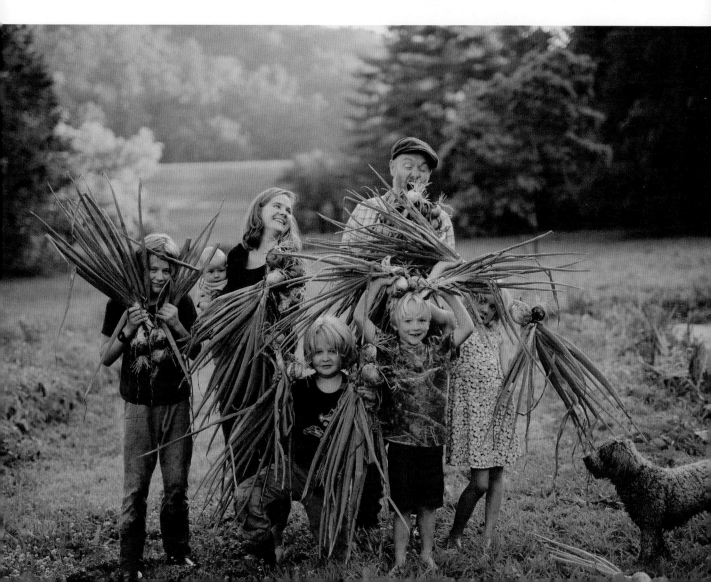

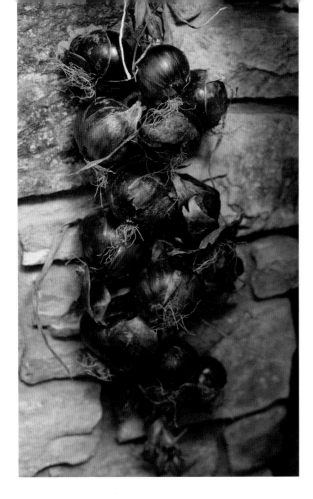

drag them back into the house for school, their hands sticky with sweetness and their faces covered in juice.

As I've been saying, having fresh produce at your fingertips that is untouched by chemicals is a huge benefit of growing your own food. Still, as you start to grow more and more, you will reach a point when you have more than you can eat. Sometimes way more! You'll reach that place of abundance, and then it will be time to figure out how to store and preserve the bounty so you can keep enjoying it once the growing season is over.

Fortunately, some foods don't need any special treatment in order to be preserved for months on end. For example:

Winter squashes. This has got to be my favorite fruit for preserving because you don't have to do much, and they can last as long as half a year on your counter at room temperature! Acorn squash and butternut squash are especially long-lasting, but spaghetti squash will go quite the distance as well.

To make this happen, it's best to let the unwashed squashes dry out a bit after harvest—this is known as curing. We built a makeshift curing rack from two-by-fours and ½-inch wire mesh. Then we just place the squashes on the rack on our covered porch for two weeks before storing them inside. Make sure there is space between them. That way if one does go bad, the rot won't spread.

Tubers. Don't wash your potatoes and sweet potatoes after the harvest—like squashes, you need to let them cure. Cure potatoes in the coolest, darkest spot you have in your house, again making sure they don't touch each other. For sweet potatoes, cure them in your greenhouse, garage, or the warmest room in your house (not touching) for two weeks. Then store in a cool, dark place.

Your tubers can touch each other after curing, so you can move them into bins or baskets after a couple of weeks. But check every now and then for any rotting spuds and remove.

Onions and garlic. Place these (not touching) on a storage rack under a shed or in your greenhouse for two weeks to cure. Then braid them in a bag and hang at room temperature.

Now, for other types of homegrown produce, when most people think of preserving, their minds automatically go to canning. After all, that's how food preservation was done for centuries.

Here's the thing, though: Rebekah and I aren't big fans of canning, and we don't can anything we grow. That's partly because you do lose some nutrients in your food when it's canned. Also, the process of canning itself is both time-intensive and nerve-racking. Things can explode, y'all!

Mostly, though, we don't can our foods because we prefer two other methods for preservation: freezing and dehydrating.

Freezing

To me, canning's biggest strength is the ability to preserve food for long periods of time without electricity. But for us grid-loving folks, the best option is freezing. That way we don't lose as many nutrients, it's not as dangerous, and we just enjoy it more.

So, here are some easy-to-use suggestions for freezing what you grow.

Veggies. We love to freeze kale and green beans, but other great freezing candidates include peas, broccoli, cauliflower, carrots, spinach, chard, collards, onions, and peppers. Herbs can also be frozen if you grow way more than you need.

To prep your veggies for the freezer, you've got to blanch them first. You do this by boiling them for three minutes, then dipping them into an ice water bath to cool them off. After a quick dip, set them out on a towel to dry. We like to vacuum-seal our veggies once they've been blanched, but you could also just bag them and freeze them.

Tomatoes. For tomatoes, we dice them, then blend them into a liquid. Then we cook them in a pot over low heat for several hours to evaporate the water. We freeze the concentrated liquidized tomatoes in meal-size freezer bags, then take them out as we need them to make tomato soup, pizza sauce, and spaghetti sauce.

Eggs. Scramble excess eggs in a bowl and pour them into a freezer bag. We like to do a dozen per bag. To cook with them later, it's best to use them in a quiche or a frittata. You could reheat them and eat them as a scramble, but the texture will be a little weird.

Meat. Freezing is a great option for all types of meat—whether chicken, turkey, beef, lamb, or pork. There are a couple of things to keep in mind. First, if you need to preserve a lot of meat, you'll need several freezers. We have seven in our household! But that's because we're big-time carnivores.

Second, remember that if you put a lot of meat in a freezer, it will take awhile for each piece to actually freeze all the way through—if everything is packed in tight, the air can't circulate. So, it's a good idea to freeze portions at a time. For example, when Rebekah and I harvest our one hundred meat chickens each season, we typically put thirty in our freezer right away. We keep the others in our walk-in cooler, and then transfer thirty more chickens to the freezer each day over the next two days. (We can get all one hundred of those chickens in a single freezer once everything is fully frozen.)

Dehydration

This is another low-key preservation method, and we love it because foods can be stored at room temperature once you're finished. Of course, you're going to need a dehydrator, and we prefer the Excalibur nine-tray model. (We replaced the stock plastic trays with stainless steel versions.) We use this often to make yogurt and to dry out nuts after soaking. This is also a great way to preserve watery vegetables such as zucchini. Just cut it into thin slices and dry them out. And check out Rebekah's recipe for dehydrated tomatoes on page 145!

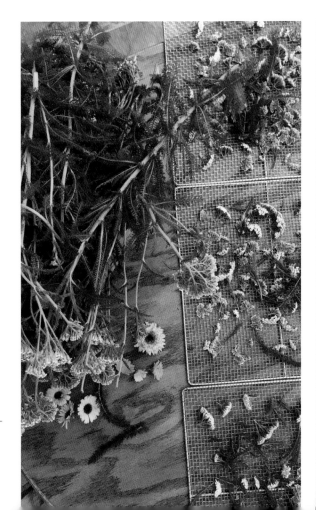

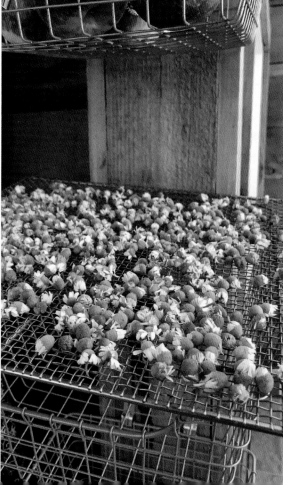

Resting Your Gardens

Remember that the growing season ends at the first frost date for your climate zone. Once that date hits and your plants have stopped producing, it's time to rest your gardens for the winter and prep them for next year's growing season.

I'll end this chapter with some step-by-step instructions for resting the three types of gardens we've focused on throughout these pages.

Container Gardens

The fastest garden to set up is also the easiest to put to rest. When each of your plants is finished producing, simply pull out the entire plant along with any weeds.

Don't empty out your containers—leave the soil right where it is. Just store the containers somewhere out of the way for the winter months and then pull them all back out again when you're ready to plant once more. If any weeds have developed over the winter storage, just pull them out before you plant.

That's it! Did I mention that Container Gardens are super easy?

One more thought. If you're using raised beds, you can put them to rest by placing a silage tarp over the top of each bed. Finish by weighing down the tarp(s) with six or eight sandbags each.

Bulletproof Gardens

This garden is almost as easy to put to rest as a Container Garden. Once again, the first thing you need to do is pull any visible weeds. And if you happen to yank out one of your plants by accident, no big deal.

The next step is to cover your garden with about 6 inches of carbonaceous material, like grass clippings, mulch, wood chips, or straw.

Then you walk away! The new layer of grass clippings or mulch will slowly turn to compost over the winter months, and you'll have healthy, fertile soil ready for planting when spring comes back around.

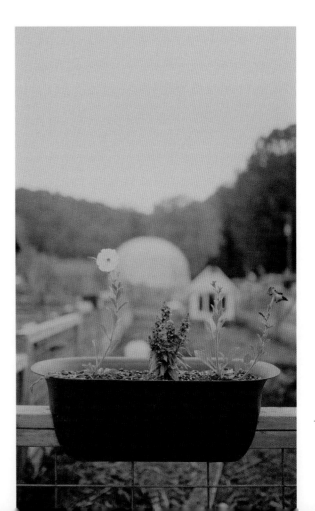

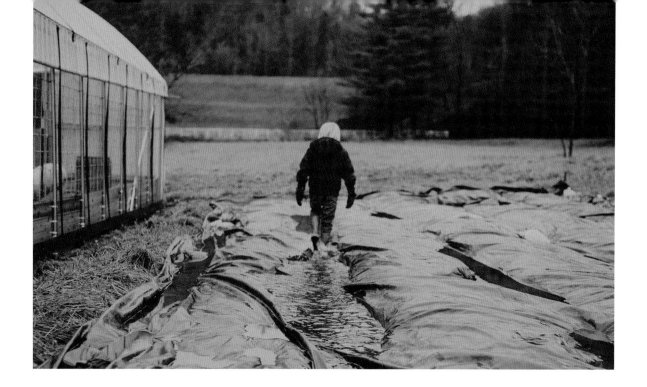

Crop Gardens

We've seen throughout these chapters that Crop Gardens require a little more work on the front end and to maintain during the growing season. That's also true when it comes to resting your Crop Gardens—but even then, the process is very simple overall.

The first step is to pull out your old crops. When your lettuces or kale or tomatoes or whatever you've grown has finished producing, just pull any remaining vegetation from the ground and leave it there to rot (as compost). No raking or digging required.

Next, remember those UV-resistant silage tarps you used to prep the garden at the very beginning and kill any remaining vegetation? Spread those bad boys back over your Crop Garden and stake them down.

Then walk away. Over the winter months, the tarps will kill any remaining vegetation, which will then become another form of compost for your soil. Those tarps will also prevent most new weeds from popping up in the spring. Last, the worms love digging around under those tarps, and they aerate the soil—not to mention adding a ton of vermicompost (worm poop), which is great for growing.

When it comes time to plant again in the spring, just pull up the tarps and plant away. You'll be ready to go.

Trust me, there's nothing quite so satisfying as harvesting food you grew yourself. I've been doing this for fifteen years, and I still get tickled by this process each year. I'm excited to see how your experiences go!

Recipes

Once you've finished harvesting and stored whatever needs to be stored, there's just one thing left to do: Eat! Feast! Enjoy! Remember, you put in all this work to grow your own food so that you and your family can have access to healthy, tasty meals at a fraction of the price. Now it's time for the payoff.

To help you enjoy your harvest even more, here are some of our favorite recipes from the Rhodes household. We hope you like them as much as we do!

The Beautiful One's Tomato Leathers

Fresh tomatoes, quartered
Salt to taste
Fresh basil to taste
Grated Parmesan cheese to taste

Blend the tomatoes in a blender or food processor.

Add as much salt, basil, and Parmesan cheese as you like.

Spread the tomato mixture across the dehydrator trays (you will need a silicone liner or parchment paper). Dehydrate at 125°F for 9 to 14 hours, depending on your region.

Cut or tear into strips. Store in a ziplock bag or jars. Enjoy!

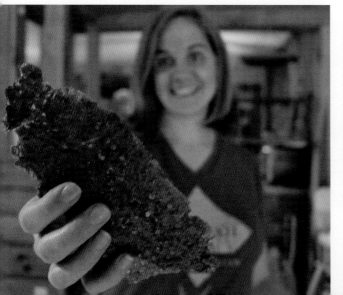
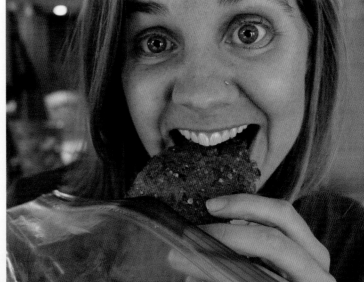

Gut-Healing Chicken Stock or Bone Broth

FOR CHICKEN STOCK

1 whole chicken

2 chicken feet (optional, but the gelatin
from them is superb)

1 chicken neck

1 chicken head (optional)

2 quarts water, or more as needed to cover
the ingredients

Veggies (optional): 2 celery stalks,
2 carrots, 2 onions, all cut in half

Salt and pepper to taste

FOR BONE BROTH

1 whole chicken carcass

2 chicken feet

1 chicken neck

1 chicken head (optional)

2 quarts water, or more as needed to cover
the ingredients

Veggies (optional): 2 celery stalks,
2 carrots, 2 onions, all cut in half

Salt and pepper to taste

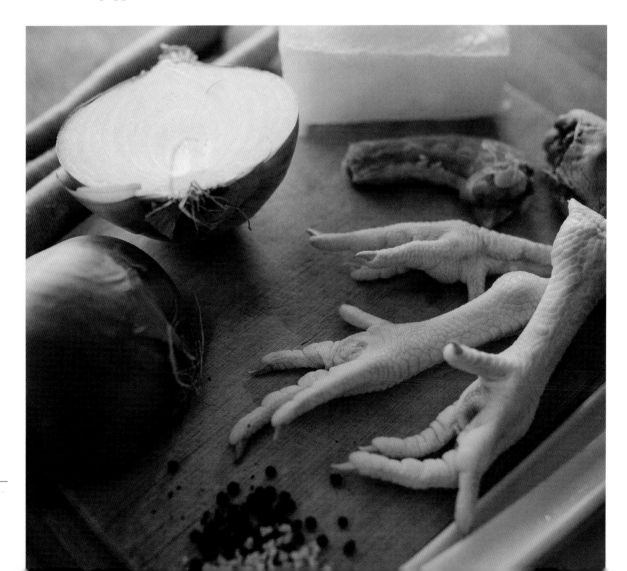

Put all the chicken parts in a gallon-size pot. Cover with water. Bring to a boil over high heat, then reduce the heat to low. Simmer for 3 hours, occasionally skimming off the crud that rises to the top.

Continue simmering for another 12 hours (good to do at night), adding water as needed to keep the bones covered.

If you're using vegetables, add them now and cook for another 5 hours, occasionally skimming off any rising crud. If you're not adding vegetables, just continue to simmer for 5-ish hours. Add water as needed to keep the bones covered.

Turn off the heat and allow to cool off for an hour or two.

Remove the large bones (and meat if you did meat stock) with tongs. Discard the bones and save the meat for another use. Get the rest of the bones, meat, vegetables, and scum with a stainless steel mesh strainer.

Set your strainer and a funnel on top of several quart or half-gallon jars and ladle your broth or stock into the jars. Close the jars and transfer to the fridge.

Heat up your desired portion in a small pot over medium heat for 5 minutes, adding salt and pepper to taste, and serve.

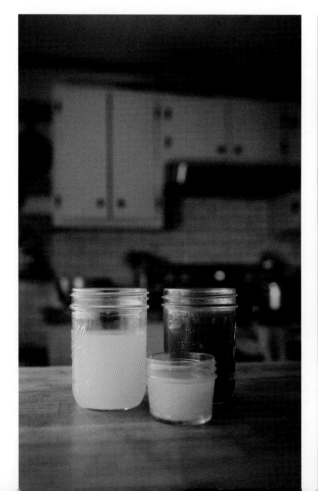
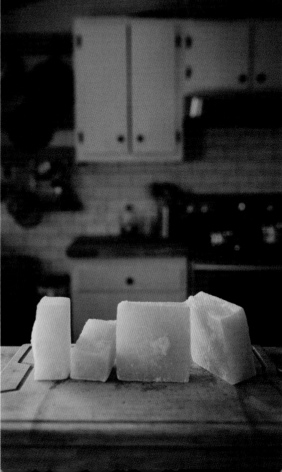

Easy Roasted Chicken

1 whole chicken, thawed
2 tablespoons butter
Salt and pepper to taste

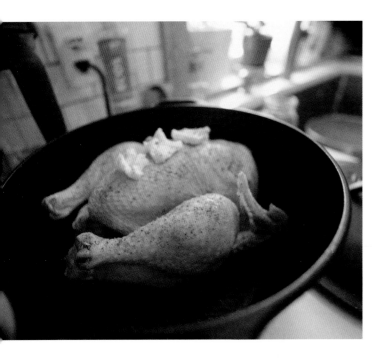

Brining is optional, but it's highly recommended if you have the time, as it will give you a nice juicy bird: Place your chicken in a large pot. Mix ½ cup salt (I like Redmond Real Salt) into 2 quarts of warm water until it dissolves. Pour the brine over the chicken, making sure the chicken is completely covered (add a little more water if necessary). Place

in the fridge until time to cook—12 hours is ideal. Remove the chicken and rinse before cooking. There's no need to season the chicken with salt before roasting as you'll have a natural salty flavor throughout. If you find it too salty or not salty enough, you can adjust the salt amount in your brine for next time.

Preheat the oven to 350°F.

Place the chicken, breast side up, on a rack in a roasting pan. (Using a rack allows heat to get to the back of the bird and keeps the chicken out of its juices. But if you don't have one, just put the chicken in the roasting pan.)

Melt the butter and brush it all over the bird. Season with pepper (and salt if you did not brine the bird).

Bake for 1½ hours, or until the temperature in the thickest part of the thigh reaches 170°F on an instant-read thermometer.

Remove from the oven and allow to sit for 30 minutes before carving.

Note: *We often roast root vegetables with the chicken so we can have a complete meal from just one pan. To do this, cut carrots, onions, and potatoes into 1- to 2-inch pieces and put in the roasting pan. Place the rack on top of the vegetables and place the chicken on the rack. The juices from the chicken will make the veggies taste fantastic!*

Justin's Classic Bacon-In Eggs

8 ounces bacon

12 eggs

Salt and pepper to taste

In a large cast-iron skillet, cook the bacon over medium heat.

Meanwhile, crack the eggs into a large bowl and season with salt and pepper. Whisk until thoroughly mixed.

Once the bacon is cooked to your liking, cut it into bite-size pieces while in the skillet.

Pour the eggs into the skillet with the bacon and bacon grease and scramble until the eggs are cooked to your liking. Serve!

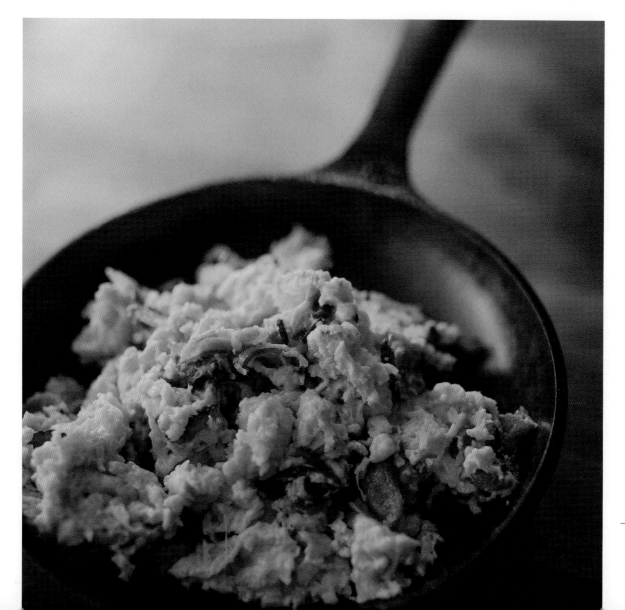

Creamy Dreamy Eggs

6 eggs

2 tablespoons heavy whipping cream

Salt and pepper to taste

2 tablespoons butter

2–4 tablespoons shredded cheddar cheese

Sliced green onions and/or diced
tomatoes, for topping (optional)

Crack the eggs into a medium bowl. Add the whipping cream and season with salt and pepper. Whisk until thoroughly combined.

Melt the butter in a cast-iron skillet over medium heat.

When the butter is melted, pour the egg mixture into the skillet and use a wooden spoon or spatula to scramble the eggs.

When the eggs are almost done, sprinkle on the cheese and mix it in so it will melt.

Top with green onions and tomatoes, if you like, and serve.

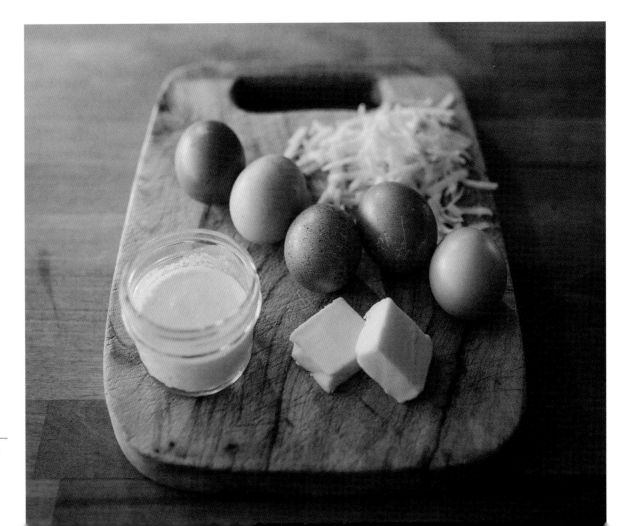

No-Carb Breakfast Casserole

1 pound loose sausage

8 ounces bacon

2 cups shredded cheddar cheese, divided

12 eggs

¾ cup heavy cream

Salt and pepper to taste

Sliced green onions, for topping (optional)

Preheat the oven to 350°F. Grease a 9 x 13-inch casserole dish. (Rubbing it down with a cold stick works great for this.)

Crumble the sausage into a large cast-iron skillet and brown well over medium heat, breaking up the meat as it cooks. Transfer the sausage to paper towels to drain the excess fat.

Add the bacon to the same skillet and cook until crisp. Transfer the bacon to paper towels to drain the excess fat. Cut or crumble the bacon into bite-size pieces.

Scatter the sausage and bacon in the prepared casserole dish. Sprinkle with 1 cup of the shredded cheese.

Crack the eggs into a medium bowl, add the cream, and season with salt and pepper. Whisk until fluffy.

Pour the eggs over the meats and cheese in the casserole dish. Sprinkle the remaining 1 cup shredded cheese over the top.

Bake for 30 minutes, or until a knife inserted in the center comes out clean.

Garnish with green onions (if using) and serve.

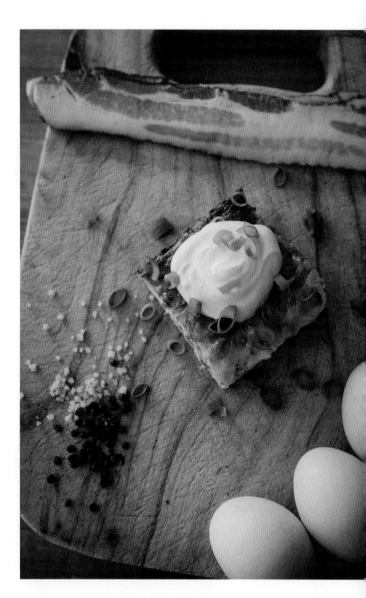

Honey-Mustard Salad Dressing

2 eggs

1 cup avocado oil (we prefer Chosen
   Foods brand)

⅓ cup honey

⅓ cup Dijon mustard

2 teaspoons lemon juice or apple cider
   vinegar

¼ teaspoon salt

Crack the eggs into a 24-ounce mason jar. Add the remaining ingredients. Using an immersion blender, blend the mixture until thickened. (If you don't have an immersion blender, you can blend everything together in a countertop blender.)

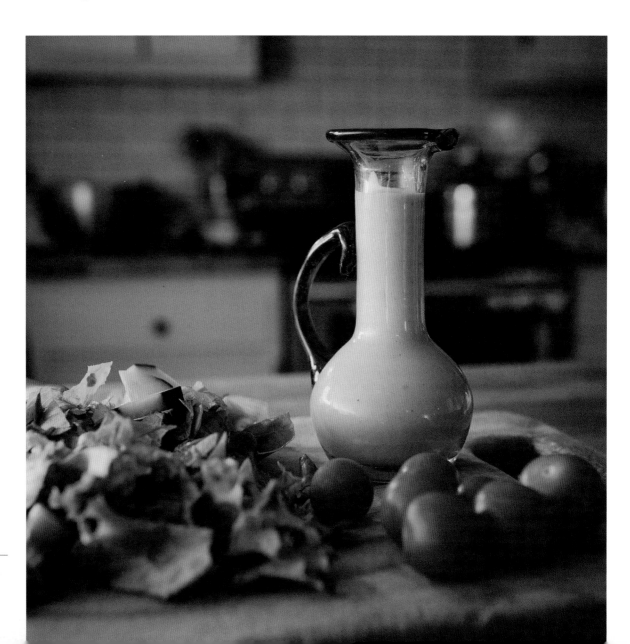

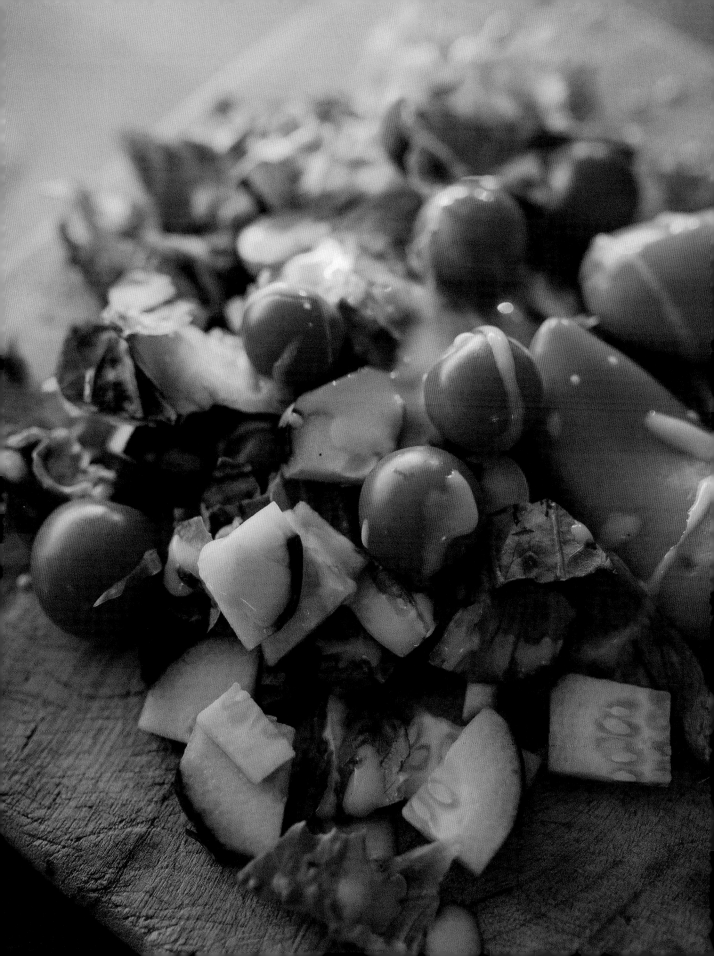

Heart (and Body) Warming Potato Soup

3 tablespoons olive oil

4–5 green onions, chopped

3–4 cloves garlic, minced

2 teaspoons dried rosemary

1 teaspoon dried parsley

1 teaspoon pepper

Salt to taste

2½ pounds red potatoes, thinly sliced

6–7 cups Chicken Stock (page 146)

1 cup milk

1–2 cups heavy cream

½ cup sour cream

Grated Parmesan cheese, for topping (optional)

Heat the olive oil in a large stockpot over medium heat. Add the green onions, garlic, rosemary, parsley, pepper, and salt and sauté until softened, about 3 minutes.

Add the potatoes and chicken stock and bring to a low boil. Cook for 15 minutes, or until the potatoes are tender.

Reduce the heat to medium-low and stir in the milk, heavy cream, and sour cream, breaking up any potatoes that might be sticking to each other. Cook until heated through.

Ladle into bowls. If desired, folks can sprinkle Parmesan cheese on top of their soup.

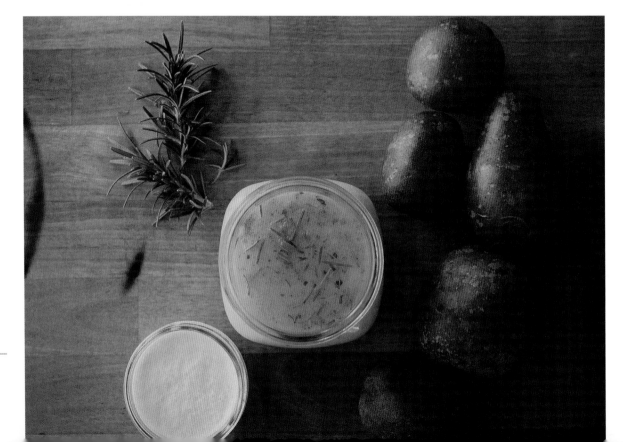

Cool, Refreshing Coleslaw

1 cup mayo

¼ cup honey

3 tablespoons lemon juice

2 tablespoons white vinegar

½ teaspoon salt

½ teaspoon pepper

½ medium cabbage, thinly sliced

2–4 carrots, grated

In a large bowl, whisk together the mayo, honey, lemon juice, vinegar, salt, and pepper.

Add the cabbage and carrots and mix until thoroughly and evenly coated in the dressing.

You can serve immediately, but for best results, refrigerate for a few hours to chill before serving.

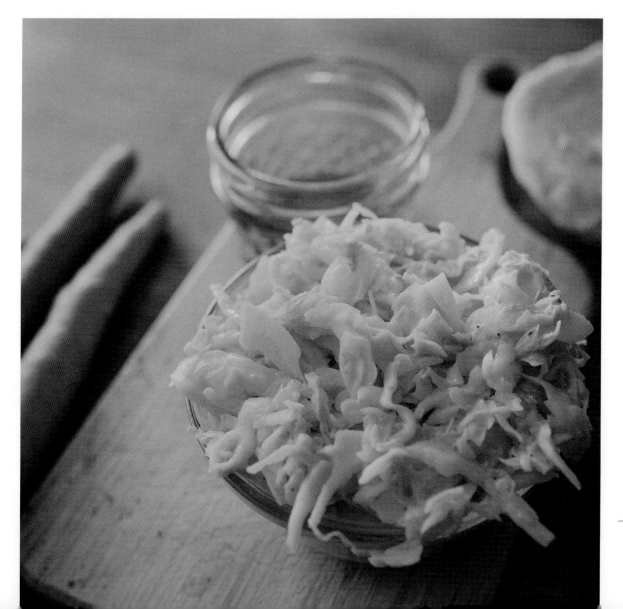

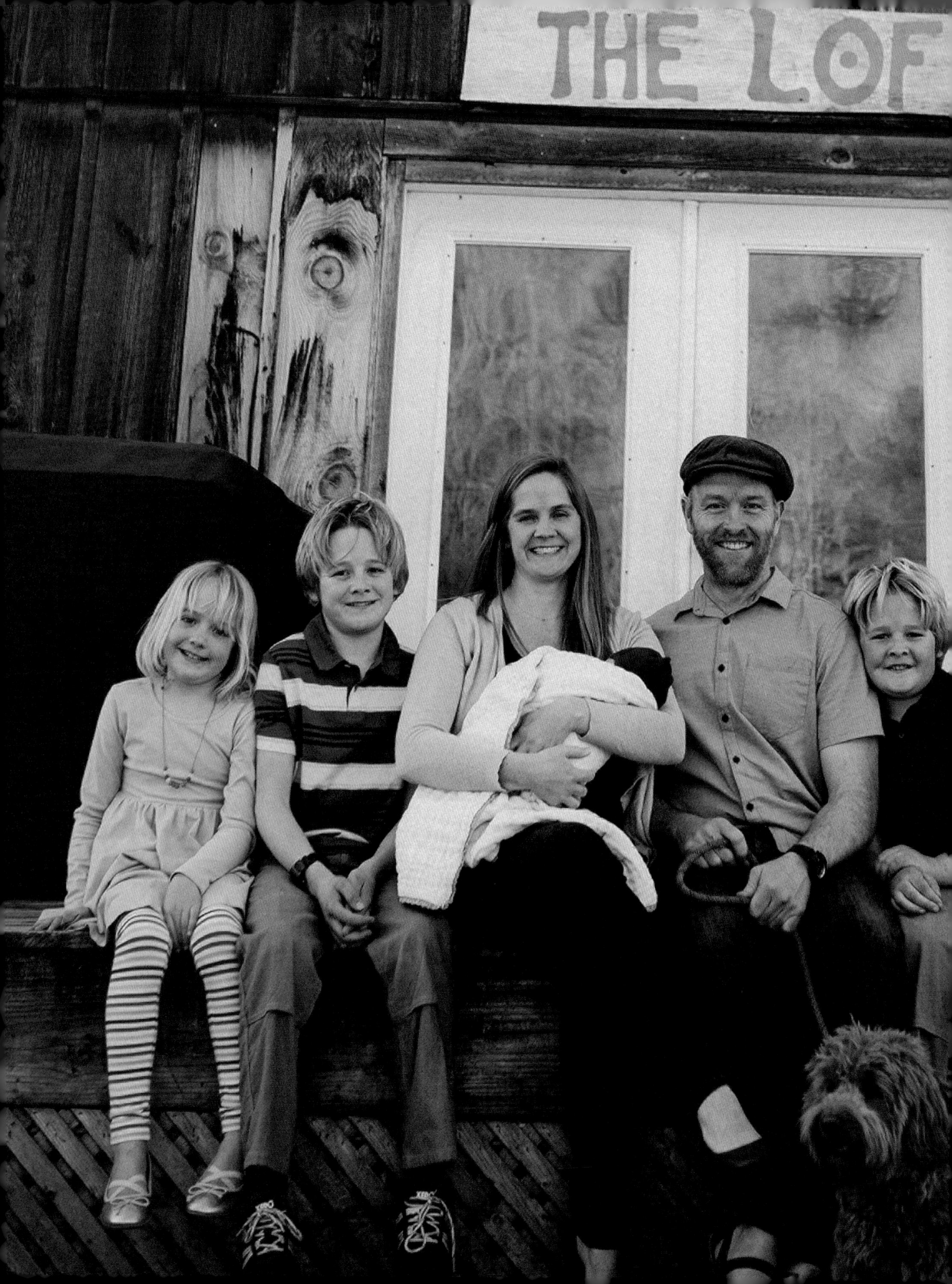
THE LOF

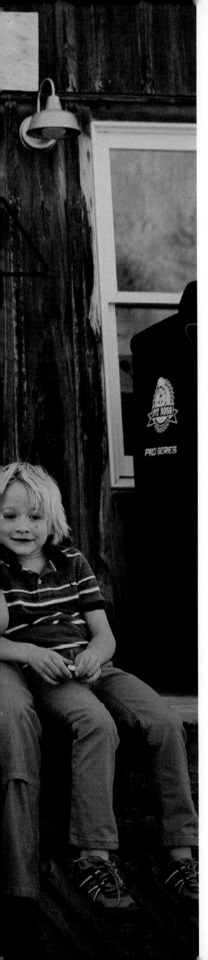

CHAPTER 9

Rooted as a Family

It happened on a regular morning, although I don't remember the day of the week. Okay, so there was a blanket of gray clouds in the sky that turned the sunrise into a muffled, muted version of itself. Sure, it was cold. And yes, it was earlier than I had planned to get up.

But it wasn't cold or darkness that overwhelmed me as I set up to milk our cows that morning. It wasn't even tiredness.

It was grief.

I was carrying two buckets through the basement when the grief washed over me, literally bringing me to my knees. I dropped the buckets, put my hands over my face, and had one of the most intense cries I've ever experienced. My shoulders shook. My breath came in sharp little bursts. I made the kind of noises you hear in movies when the actor is really hamming it up to show how wrecked he's feeling after some twist in the plot.

This was during the period of my life when I was trying to figure out how to make our homestead work despite the symptoms that had crashed down over me through my chronic Lyme disease. Emotionally, I was drained and empty. Mentally, I had trouble keeping up with everything that needed to be processed and performed. Physically, I felt like I couldn't take another step.

And I really did hate milking those cows. Getting up early all by myself morning after morning and trudging through the darkness to sit with a couple of cows just wasn't fun. It was my least favorite chore.

So yeah, I cried for a long time. The question that kept knocking around in my brain was frustrating, given that I had no answer: *How in the world can I keep this up?*

Well, I eventually cried myself out and got off my knees. I milked the cows that morning and the morning after. And the morning after that. I continued to drag myself forward, while at the same time I learned new methods of treatment for my illness, and Rebekah and I learned new ways to make our homestead and our lives more manageable. Time worked its magic on my wounds.

Then, just about a year ago, something else happened that caught my attention. I was milking cows again—another cold, early morning. But this time my boy Jonah—my oldest—was with me. We were laughing and cutting up a little bit when he asked me a question out of the blue.

"Dad, do you like milking cows?"

"Yes," I said. "I love it."

Then I stopped. I'd spoken without thinking, but I realized in that moment that I'd told my son the truth. I truly did love milking the cows. In fact, I milked those cows this morning, and I still love it!

I thought to myself, *What changed?* The answer was my children. They've grown up a bit in recent years, which means one or more of them come with me when I do just about anything on our homestead. Yes, they can pitch in with the physical tasks, which is helpful. But much more importantly, they pitch in *with me.* They talk with me, laugh with me, and just spend time with me.

My children have become my companions. And their friendship has become the difference between grief and joy.

That's what I want to focus on in this chapter, because pursuing the rooted life is more than just growing food or getting healthy or saving money. The rooted life is about cultivating abundance and wellness and joy. It's about peace and purpose—the element of *life* is critical.

Rebekah and I don't invest our time in this journey just to grow corn or cabbages or eggs or beef. We're growing children. We're growing a family. And we want to help you do the same.

So, what you'll find here are some of our best tips and tricks for bringing the whole family on board as you work together to grow all the goodness you can harvest.

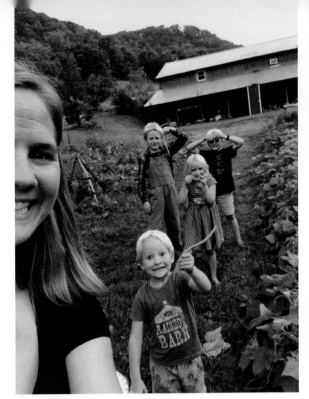

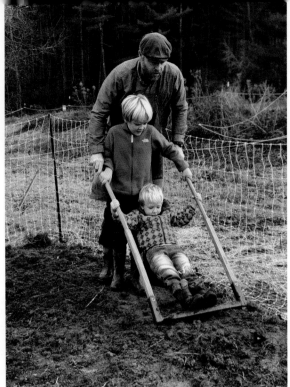

How to Get Your Children Involved

Growing up, my dad would occasionally take me or one of my siblings along with him on orthodontics sales calls. That was about as exciting as it sounds. Now that I have my own children, I feel for those office workers who, no doubt, ended up babysitting us in the waiting room while Dad called on the doctors.

One time there was a pretty receptionist who tried to engage me in conversation by asking, "Hey there, little guy, do you like traveling with your dad?"

To which I flatly responded, "No. He farts too much."

Over my entire life, I've never seen my dad so embarrassed! In fact, up to the day he died, he still blushed whenever I brought up the way I hung his dirty laundry in front of that young lady.

All that is to say, I'm glad there's no such thing as "Bring Your Kids to Work Day" in our family. On our homestead, that's just Tuesday! And Wednesday. And Thursday. And so on. Of course, it's not always easy. There's some work (and maybe a little magic) involved with getting our kids to participate. But they do participate, and it's always worth it.

So, here are some tips and tricks Rebekah and I have picked up along the way that will hopefully help you achieve the same thing.

Want Them and Invite Them

The best thing you can do to get your kids involved with the rooted life is to invite them.

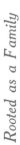

That's it. I've seen it work countless times—with our kids, yes, but also many others. Children will often be inspired to follow you if you simply ask them to.

It may help to be creative with that invitation. Being persistent, begging, or even bribing may be necessary (more on that below). But in the end, just letting your kids know that you want to spend time with them and asking them to join you will go a long way toward gaining you some companions as you work to grow your own food.

Help Them Get Started

This is especially true for younger chiddlers. As parents, it's easy for us to focus on the growth we want our kids to experience by pitching in with chores. "It's good for them. It builds character!" That certainly can be true,

but it's also necessary for us to help them get started in that process.

Help your kids get dressed, for example. Find their shoes. Make them a snack. Do whatever you can to make the overall experience as easy and as positive as possible.

This is something I used to struggle with quite a bit. My son Mr. Brown is the world's worst when it comes to keeping track of his shoes. He can lose tennis shoes, Crocs, boots, or any other footwear in a flash. But, that's a lesson for another day. Right now I want him to be with me, so our first step in going outside is a father-son search for his shoes. And that's okay. He's coming outside to "help" me, so I can return the favor by helping him get started. I try to constantly remember that he'll soon grow up and find his own shoes, which means I need to treasure the frustrations

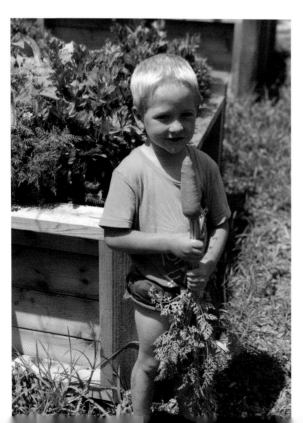

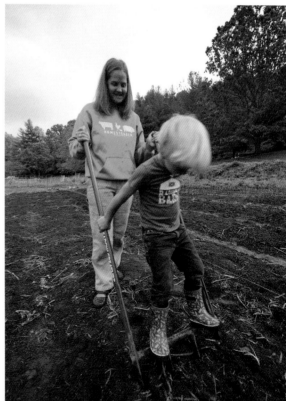

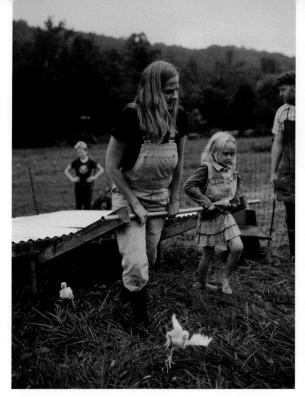

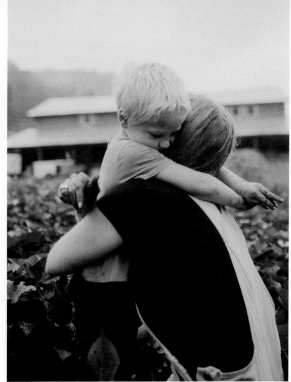

of working with my young children while they last.

Let Them Help

When you invite your children to help with your chores, they will naturally want to pitch in—which may mean they want to do things they're not really ready to do, or things you would rather do yourself. That means you need patience. Yes, I understand you could toss out that chicken food about ten times faster than your little apprentice, but that's not really the point. Right?

Remember, you're growing chiddlers, not just food. When you put your kids on the "to-do" list, quality time becomes the agenda rather than a side benefit.

To give you an example, I create a lot of vlogs for our YouTube channel. People often

ask me if the camera gets in the way, and the answer is yes. It slows me down maybe 15 or 25 percent. That's why I constantly remind myself we're not just out doing chores, we're out making a movie about doing chores. When the filmmaking becomes the priority, suddenly it's no longer "in the way." The same is true with letting your chiddlers help.

Now here's the trick: When you're planning to do some chore with your little ones, just plan on it taking 25 percent longer than if you did it yourself. Account for that on the front end, by either giving yourself more time or aiming to do less. That will go a long way toward calming your nerves.

Let Them Fail

As parents, we're constantly afraid that our children will mess up. I've found this fear is

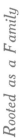

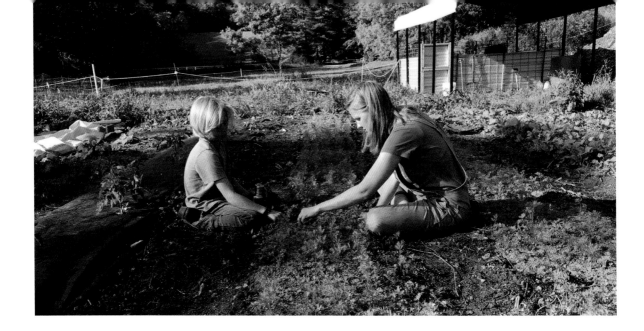

especially prevalent when I've invested time and money in something—such as growing my own food.

Well, spoiler alert: They will fail. So will you. But that's why you should plant or plan to grow 25 percent more than you need. That way you won't get so upset if the chiddlers stomp on those young cabbages and crush them. Or drop those eggs coming in from the chicken house.

If it's emotionally and physically possible, I encourage you to let your children experiment. Let them have their own section of the garden to work as they please. The worst thing that can happen is that their garden gets overrun with weeds and produces no harvest. On the flip side, the best thing that can happen— whether they succeed or fail—is that they remember how Mom and Dad had their backs and supported them. Also, if they fail, you then have the chance to comfort them. "You did your best. What did you learn?"

Here's something to think about, though: you might be surprised by what your kids come up with that actually *works*.

One day we were all out planting a garden when Jonah asked if he could plant his own garden in a certain area. I said sure and let him go at it. I committed in my heart to be there for him, but not to direct him in any way unless he asked. Well, after a few minutes

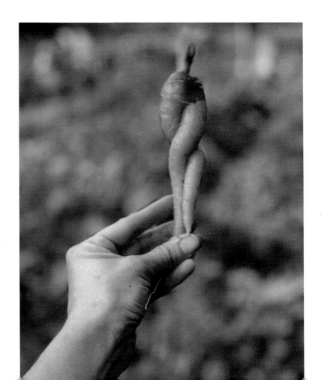

I looked over and noticed he was planting waaaaaay too many seeds in his little area. There was no way it could work. Still, as hard as it was, I didn't say anything except maybe, "Good job, let's hope for the best."

Ha! Turns out reality had a little lesson for me. No lie, Jonah's patch ended up performing better than the rest of our garden. The seeds actually benefited from being planted so close together because the close-growing plants crowded out any weeds, and the taller plants gave shade for his lettuces (which happen to like a little shade). From that point on, we haven't been afraid to break the rules and experiment, especially with plant spacing.

For older children, allowing them to fail means letting out the reins (which can be terribly hard) and letting them take over larger responsibilities—even though it might not turn out well. Failure needs to be not just allowed, but part of the learning process. That said, you can certainly encourage them to fail small. When they have an exciting idea, be careful about speaking your wisdom. Even if you know it's not going to work, hold your tongue and let them go for it (unless they're going to hurt themselves or someone else).

Basically, choose to leave a legacy as a cheerleader, not a dream crusher. No one ever speaks fondly of their late parents by saying, "Boy, I'm glad they held me back." No, you want them to say, "They supported me no matter what."

Give Them Their Own Chores

Everybody loves having responsibilities according to their skill level, including young people. For example, our ten-year-old daughter, Lily, is responsible for the chickens in the front yard. It's not hard, it's not dangerous, and she seems to enjoy the birds. Plus, the work she

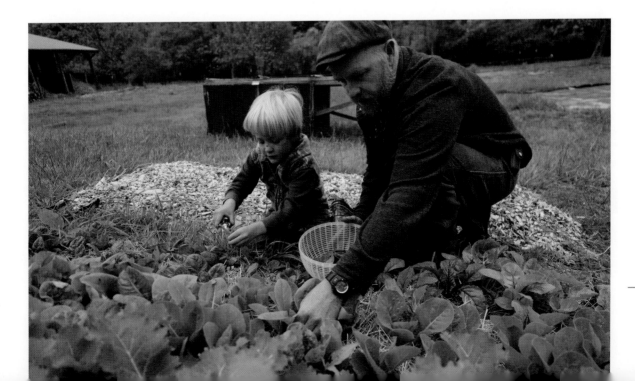

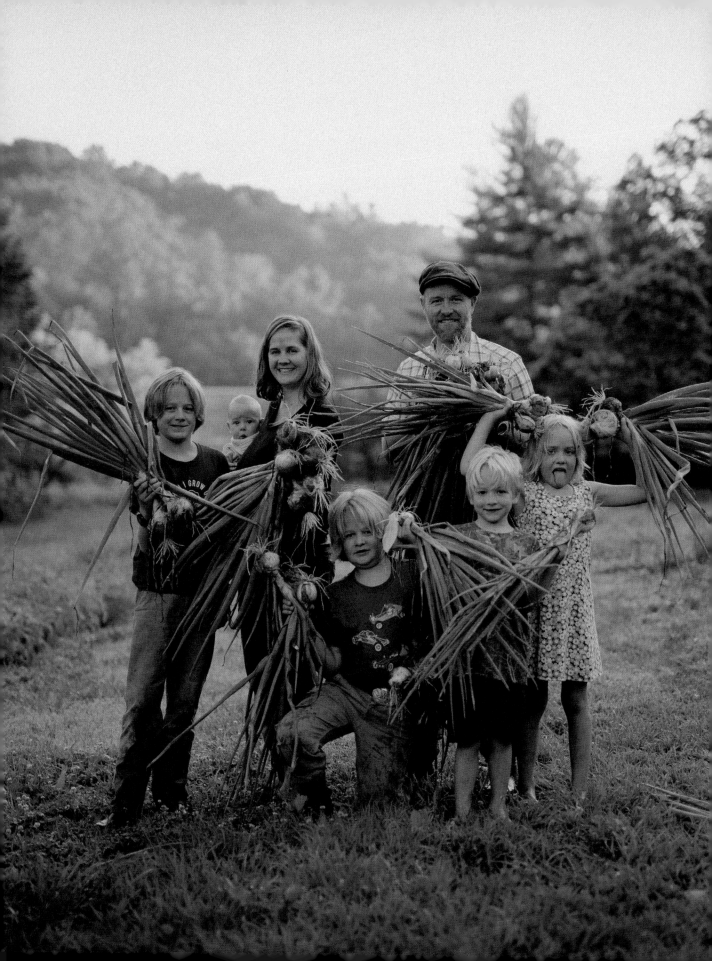

does is legitimately helpful for our operation, which is an added bonus.

We've found that what children like or dislike can play a critical role in assigning chores. Whenever possible, we try to cater to those preferences. For instance, Jonah can't stand milking cows, but Lily loves it. So, Lily joins me every morning for the milking, and then Jonah is (mostly) happy to move the cows over to a new paddock or take on another more exciting role.

We haven't quite hit this stage yet, but I know Joel Salatin has had great success allowing his son Daniel to take responsibility for new and different elements on their farm. Over time, Daniel has taken more and more responsibility, even to the point where the leadership roles have actually switched. Now, Joel asks Daniel what to do. Hopefully it will be the same for me one day!

Ask Their Opinion—Then Try It!

Making decisions is part of what it means to be human. Unfortunately, that's an opportunity that many chiddlers are denied, especially when they're young. For kids, other people make *all* the decisions, and they often long for the moment when their opinion will matter and they get to make a choice.

As a parent, we can give our kids those opportunities as part of our journey toward the rooted life. Imagine a moment when you're out there working with your little ones, and you come to a fork in the road. Both options look okay. Why not ask a child which one you should take? Get their opinion. And then—just as important—do what they suggest. (Within reason, of course.)

Your children will thrive when they get some opportunities to decide. With that in mind, here are some great beginnings to good questions:

- Should we…?
- Why do you think…?
- What would happen if we…?
- What do you think about…?

Make It Quality Time

When it comes to your family, time together is time together. Period. Despite popular belief, quality time doesn't have to be a superfun day at Go Kart Land. Quality time can be solving real-world problems together in the front yard.

As I mentioned earlier, my ten-year-old daughter, Lily, milks cows with me every single morning. That's twenty to forty minutes of work, rain or shine, seven days a week—including her birthday. Christmas too. If you ask her, she'll tell you she likes it. I happen to believe her, but I don't think it's all about milking. I think being with me goes a long way toward making those moments more than a chore.

That's one of the key values and benefits of the rooted life: Simply working together. Doing something good side by side.

If you want to take things to the next

level, ask questions while you work. Ask your chiddlers about what's happening in their day and their lives. Ask them what they like or don't like. Ask for their opinions about things. Tell them stories. Ask them to tell you stories. As they begin to talk, you'll soon find plenty more questions that come naturally. When it goes silent, don't sweat it. Expressions of love and affection don't always include words, and often a tight bond can be formed by just silently working together on the same thing.

Here are some specific ideas for turning chore time into quality time:

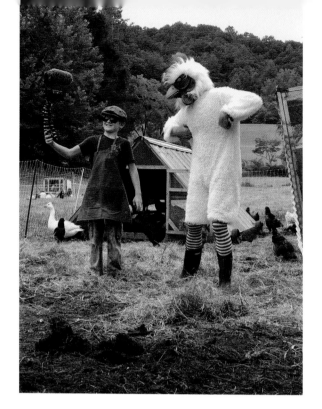

- Have certain chores you do with certain children (based on their preference).
- Take turns doing the chores with each child while giving the others a break.
- Take turns bringing children to town on errands or long trips.
- Take turns having children help you cook.

Let Them Play

Another way to involve your young ones in the rooted life is to invite them along without requiring that they "chip in." This is especially important for young children who are still primarily interested in playing, perhaps twelve or younger. Here's why this makes sense: Your child will likely be excited about transplanting plants in the garden at first, but they will soon get bored. Perhaps you've set up a reward if they finish, or not. Either way, giving them the

option to either keep helping or start playing has benefits.

What's the benefit of letting them play? They're having fun! They're associating being outside with you and engaging the land with something good and enjoyable.

I've talked with lots of folks who grew up on homesteads but dreaded every moment. Why? Because they were forced to work a lot of hours and given very little time to play. And when they did play, it was by themselves or with siblings. They were separated from their parents, who were busy working.

For the Rhodes family, we want to build an association between farming and having fun. That farming means being around Mom and Dad. Because we believe that in the long term, such an association will lead them to take on more responsibility.

An Urgent Message to Dads

I'd like to say something specifically to fathers for just a moment. Dads, remember, there's no rule for what you can and cannot do with your children. There are no regulations about what is "manly" and what is "womanly." There's just stuff that needs to get done and people who need to do it.

For example, I wake up our chiddlers and take them with me on farm chores. I cook them breakfast. I help with homeschooling. I take them on town trips. I take them on long trips. I take them practically everywhere with me. Not just to the farm, but to the bank or the hardware store. If I had a "regular" job in an office, they'd go with me there, too, as much as possible. And if they weren't allowed to come, I'd find another job—or, better yet, create my own job at home as an entrepreneur.

Society has a dream for you, but that doesn't mean it's your dream. You can dream your own dreams, make up your own rules, and live your own life. It's time to shake off any social, political, or even religious stigmas you may be carrying and take a stand for yourself and your family. Opt out of any selfish or societal pressure to behave in a specific way. Step up to the plate and be the father you know you want to be—and the father your children so desperately need.

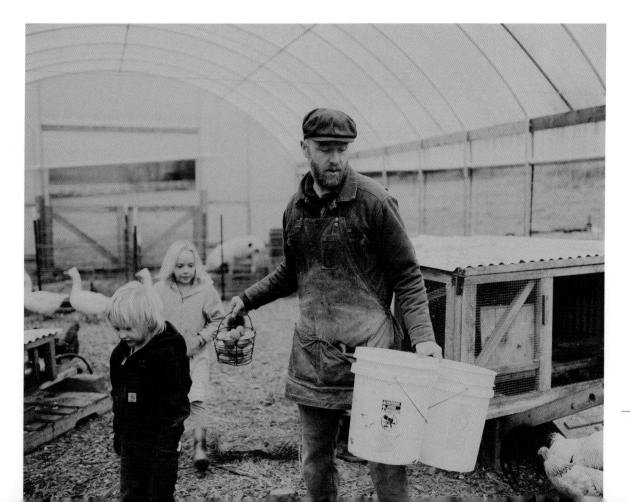

How to Work Closely with Your Spouse
(Without Killing Each Other)

Rebekah and I were driving down the road on our first date in over a year. Our oldest child, Jonah, was finally at the age where we could leave him with a babysitter for an hour or two, and we were taking advantage. We were excited! Well, I was excited. Rebekah was a bit anxious about leaving our baby.

As we drove, I found myself captivated by the North Carolina scenery. So much to see! No babies crying. No chickens to feed or cows to milk. I was just digging the road, the view, and the silence.

That's when Rebekah started sharing about her emotions. She talked about the guilt she was feeling. She told me there was a lot of fear in her heart. She knew intellectually that Jonah would be fine, he would probably sleep the whole time we were gone. But she couldn't help this nagging idea that—

"Look, Rebekah!" I blurted out, my voice filled with both horror and glee. "Shirtless Man is throwing hay without a shirt!"

Okay, a little background. Rebekah and I have a neighbor who almost never wears a shirt. Well, it's rural North Carolina, so you get used to some things. We call him Shirtless Man. But that day, as we were driving along, I happened to look over and see this particular gentleman throwing hay in his yard still without a shirt! If you've never dealt with hay, it's incredibly itchy. It gets everywhere and just digs right into your skin. I would never try to throw hay in short sleeves, let alone *no shirt at all!*

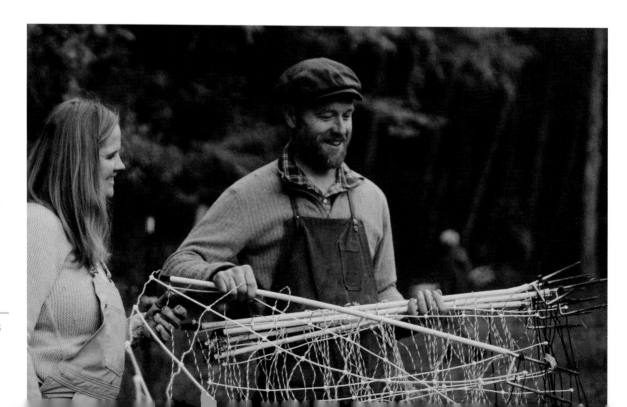

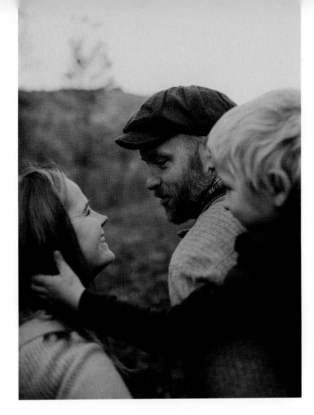

I looked over at Rebekah to see the look on her face when she realized how funny this situation was. "Can you believe…?" Oh. Not the look I was counting on. Not even close.

Turns out I should have been listening to my wife pour out her heart rather than goofing off about our shirtless neighbor, humorous or not. I apologized, and thankfully we were able to push through and have a great time on that first date.

I tell that story because the rooted life doesn't impact only the relationships between parents and children. It takes a lot of work to grow your own food, especially if you are growing a significant amount. More than likely, that means you and your spouse will be sharing the majority of that work—which means you'll be working together more than you might have anticipated.

You know what Rebekah and I have found? Working with your spouse on something as big as growing your own food is much different from simply *living* with your spouse. There's a different kind of relationship that develops—or that needs to develop if you're going to succeed.

So, we'd like to share just a few tips we've learned for pursuing the rooted life with your spouse in a way that maximizes your relationship, rather than causing extra strain.

Find Time for Each Other

It's always important to continue "dating" your spouse as a married couple. You were together before your kids came along, and you'll likely be together long after they are gone, so it's important to maintain that relationship throughout. But it's even more important to make social time for each other when you spend a lot of time working together.

Sure, it can be very hard to get away from home. Believe me, I know. But you don't have to get away to be together. These days when Rebekah and I hire a babysitter, we often stay home while the babysitter takes the kids outside!

Even if you can't have an actual date, you can find time at home alone. We used to do that after the children went to bed. Now that they're growing older and don't go to bed as early, Rebekah and I have to be more creative. We go on walks or get up early for a little "us time." Actually, one of the best things we've done for our health and marriage was to get a two-seater sauna. Every night, we look forward to sitting together for forty minutes just detoxing, chatting together, resting, or reading books. Even if we're not actively talking with each other, we're still together.

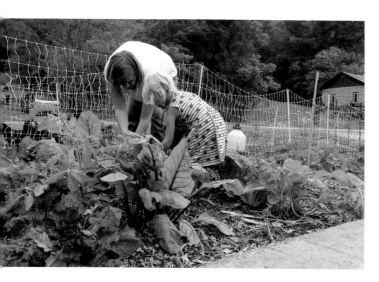

The point is, it takes work to pursue the rooted life. And if you've got "day jobs," that work can feel like something extra. Another spinning plate. But be absolutely certain you don't make time for that work by whittling away time with your spouse. That relationship is just too important.

Communicate and Listen

Duh, right? What else can I add? I mean, there are entire collections of books dedicated to this idea within relationships.

The only thing I'll say here is that communication in marriage is always hard,

and it doesn't get easier just because you spend more time together. (Actually, sometimes that can make things harder.) Even if you spend hours in close proximity each week preparing seed starts or weeding in the garden, you still need to put in the effort for effective communication.

This is difficult for me because I'm a *bad* listener. Even in the middle of a conversation, I'll start daydreaming or working on ideas in my brain. Sometimes I'll even ask Rebekah a question, then zone out right away and not even pay attention to the answer! It can be a real struggle in our marriage. (Remember the Shirtless Man?)

Thankfully, I've learned I can make up for my bad listening with good talking. And that's really one of the secrets to my marriage with Rebekah. We talk about everything! We tell each other everything. We share thoughts, fears, emotions, and more. That includes being honest when we're feeling hurt, and that includes a lot of apologizing. Mostly from me. (Remember the Shirtless Man?)

One of the best things Rebekah and I have done for our marriage is to go to bed at the same time. Once the kids have finally gone to bed, we'll follow suit. I'll grab her hand and we'll quietly talk about our hopes, dreams, and certainly our frustrations. Sometimes, I'll even get lucky. (Which is also an important part of maintaining and strengthening any marriage. Right?)

Walk in Each Other's Forgiveness

One of my mentors, Mark Lucas, spoke these words of advice at his wife's funeral. He said the key to a good relationship is to understand that we all fail. We just have to walk in each other's forgiveness. Isn't that powerful?

I've seen entire marriages end because one spouse wouldn't apologize or go to marriage counseling. It's hard to admit when we've failed, and it can be super hard to forgive someone as close as a spouse when they mess up. Again, this doesn't get easier just because you're growing food together.

The way Rebekah and I deal with our failures is to apologize. I'm very quick to apologize, probably to a fault. Sometimes it comes across as cheap, and sometimes it probably is. Rebekah's not as quick, but when she does apologize it's sweeter. But we've

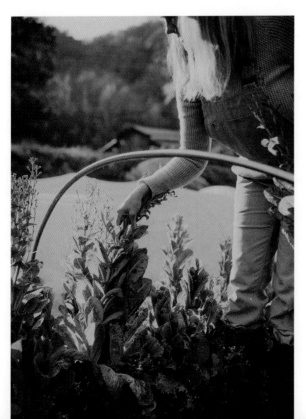

chosen to walk in each other's forgiveness. We talk to each other *knowing* that forgiveness is available.

Now, sometimes we do seek out those apologies. If I've hurt my wife and am refusing to talk about it, she'll come to me and ask for an apology. She'll tell me why she needs one, and usually I see exactly what she means by the time she's finished. And the blessing for me is that I can apologize, knowing that forgiveness will be there.

Sometimes we have to walk away, take breaks, or sleep on it. (Yes, we occasionally go to bed angry.) Sometimes we text each other even if we're in the same room. Actually, texting can be helpful because it's impossible to raise your voice, and you get to make sure you say what you mean.

The point is, we revisit the issue until we work it out. Given the amount of time we spend together, I know if we just shove away the hurt and try to bury it, everything will just accumulate and eventually explode. So we choose the other path. We choose to talk it out and walk in each other's forgiveness rather than in our own selfish pride.

Play to Each Other's Strengths

It's no secret that people think differently on an individual level, and most people who are married have noticed that men and women often think differently on a general level. Those differences can be a source of conflict, but they can also be a source of strength!

What Rebekah and I have found over the years is that we can support each other *and* do a better job of reaching our goals when we exploit each other's strengths rather than weaknesses. Meaning, I can lean on her strengths and allow her to shine in those areas rather than focusing on her weaknesses and trying to get her to improve. (And vice versa, of course.)

For example, one of our biggest issues early in our marriage was the way we presented our ideas to each other. Rebekah tends to think things through before presenting new ideas to me. I tend to present my ideas before I think them through; it's part of my creative process. Neither of those approaches is wrong—they're just different. But we didn't know that about each other at first.

So, when I'd blurt out some ridiculous idea that just came into my head, Rebekah would lose her mind because she figured I'd put a bunch of thought into this—it must be something I really wanted to do—but she was seeing all kinds of problems. Out of fear, she would aggressively shoot down the idea and maybe even feel offended that I would seriously consider something so absurd. (When in truth I wasn't considering it much at all; it just popped into my head.)

Over time, we've come to realize that our differences make us stronger. Rebekah can make connections I never see. And she can think of things at a level of depth that's difficult for me. So, she is an ideal sounding board. When I have an idea, I just start firing things her way. If it's a good idea, she helps me go deeper. If it's a bad idea, she helps me see the flaws, and I can move on.

How to Get Your Spouse on Board

This may come as a surprise, but this whole homestead thing was not my idea. In fact, *none of it* was my idea. Chickens. Gardens. Cows. None of it. It was Rebekah who started doing the research on the benefits of eating healthier. It was Rebekah who started thinking about expanding our operations, using more of our land, starting market gardens, and so on. I was supportive, but she was the driving force.

Things took a turn when she got pregnant with our second child, Josiah, and experienced terrible morning sickness. That's when I started taking a far more active role in the planning and execution of our homestead. But it was a gradual process.

My heart goes out to anyone seeking to live a more rooted life *without* the support of their significant other. That's tough. But I'm also a living example that things can change. So, here are a few thoughts on how you can handle things if you are excited about growing your

The Rooted Life

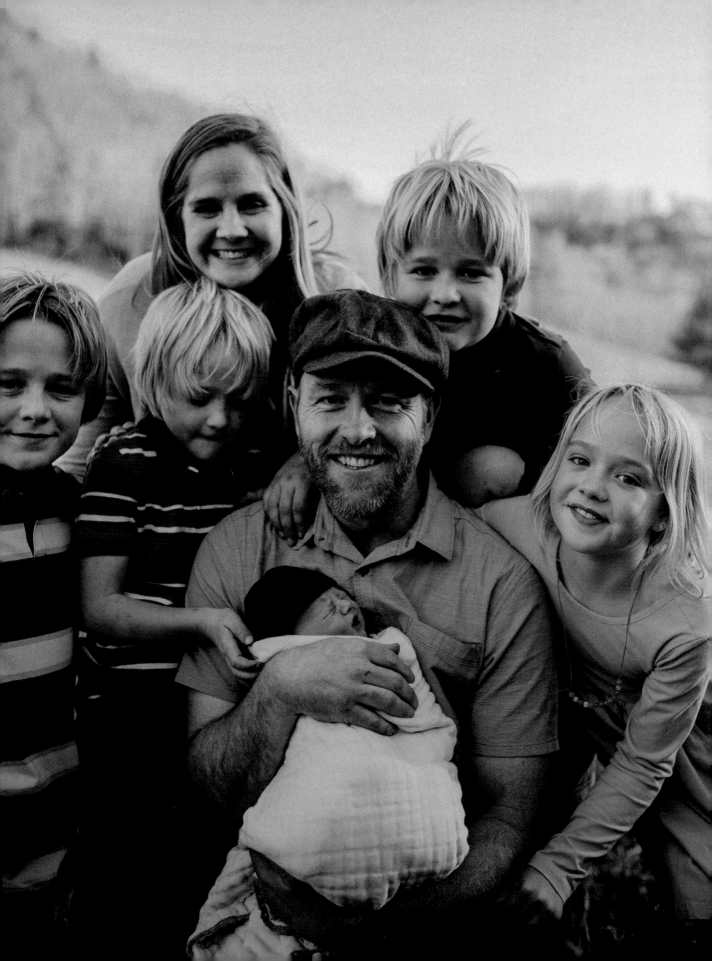

own food and you'd like to get your partner on board.

Support Them Anyway

First and foremost, you need to come to grips with the reality that they may never get on board—and that's okay. I'm serious. I know that's not the answer you're looking for, but relationships are more important than a specific type of lifestyle. So, even if your spouse never comes around, support them anyway.

Think about it from their perspective. Living a more rooted life probably wasn't on either of your radars when you committed to each other, and it's usually a *big* change. So you can't expect to snap your fingers and have them see things the same way you do.

Plus, there's the simple fact that you can't change your spouse's perspective or beliefs. Instead, I say meet them where they're at and support them in their own interests. Who

knows what might happen when you start putting them first? There's a natural sense of softening that comes from reciprocity. Help them get what they want from life, and they will be more likely to help you in this new way of life.

Start Small

Of course, just because your spouse isn't on board doesn't mean you should delay your own goals. You can start moving yourself toward a more rooted way of life, and you can ask the other members of your family to follow as much as they're comfortable.

When you do get going, I suggest you start small. Move slowly. Make sure pushing toward the rooted life doesn't have a negative impact on your relationships, and listen to what your partner thinks. If your spouse really doesn't want to deal with chickens in the yard, that should mean no chickens—at least for now.

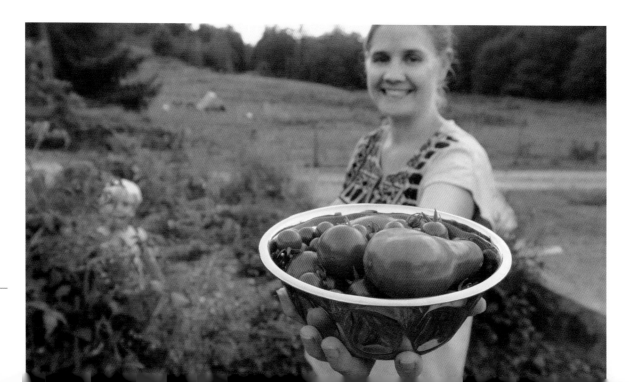

Stick with gardens and give your spouse some time to come around.

One good trick is to share what makes you excited. When you have a victory—that first harvest is always a great example—share it with your spouse. Share your feelings too. Talk about how good it feels (and how good it tastes!) to grow something and be part of the story.

Bribe Them

There's nothing wrong with a good bribe between spouses! So if you're going to take some initial steps toward growing your own food, start by growing what your spouse loves. If you've got a little garden growing and they love Greek salads, give them the best, freshest, tastiest Greek salad you can muster.

Honestly, this works. Sometimes the best way to a person's heart is through their belly.

Also, be active in inviting your spouse to participate in the fun stuff. Letting the chickens out is fun, for example. Harvesting berries is a ton of fun. Your goal here is to whet their appetite by showing that growing your own food isn't just work—there's a lot of reward involved.

Keep things low pressure. "Hey darling, would you like to go for a walk and see what I've grown?" Invite them to be excited with you.

I want to repeat what I said at the beginning of this chapter because I think it's critical: The rooted life is not a method for growing food. It's not even a prescription for a healthier life. (Although food and health are a critical part of what it means to be more rooted.)

No, the rooted life is a choice to seek abundance in your life and in the lives of your loved ones. It's a decision to cultivate *wellness* in every sense of that word.

Yes, I hope you continue down this path of growing your own food. Yes, I hope you grow a ton of wonderful things and enjoy that bounty all year long. And yes, I would like to be with you in the process and teach you as much as you'd like to learn.

But my biggest hope is that you and I and millions like us will grow healthy families so that we can work together to change the world in big ways.

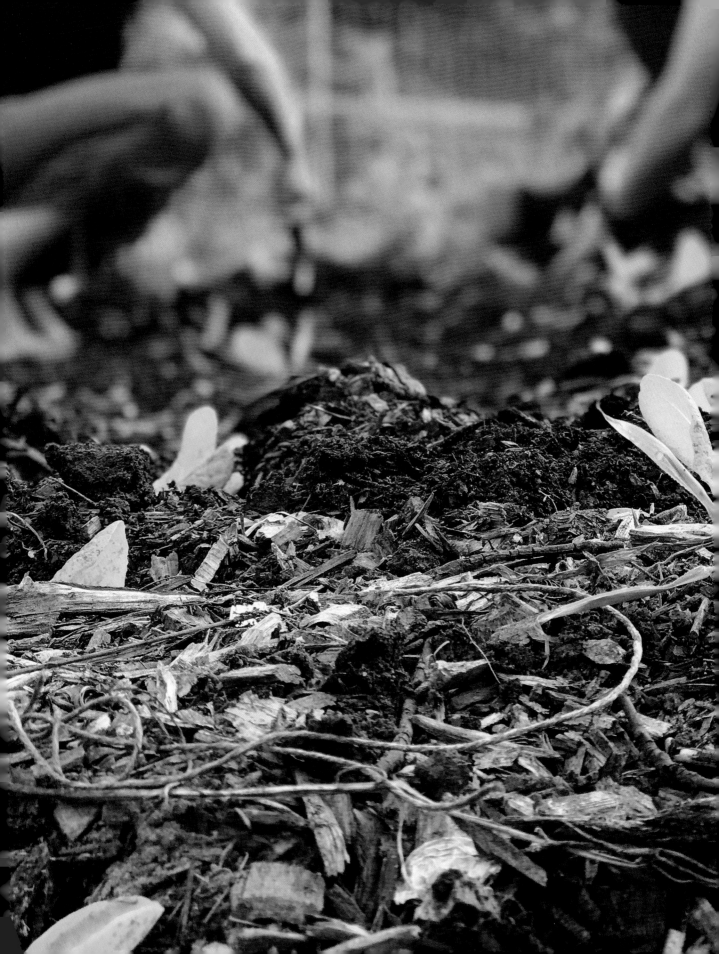

CHAPTER 10

Just Plant !

Back in 2016, Rebekah and I started our first "100 Days of Growing Food" challenge. This was in the early days of our YouTube channel, and we wanted to see how much food we could grow from start to finish in just a hundred days, with our family working only about ten hours a week.

Mind you, this was starting from scratch. We didn't use any of our existing gardens. We didn't use any of our existing chicken flocks. We did everything from scratch.

We started in May, and we concentrated on gardens and chickens. We worked through that growing season, and we were surprised to find that we could grow around 75 percent of our food without stretching over that ten hours a week. And this was on only about half an acre.

The experiment was a huge success for us personally, and it was a big hit on our channel. When that hundred days came to a close, we knew we needed to celebrate in some way. That's when Rebekah had an idea: "Why don't we invite people to come celebrate with us? We could have a potluck!"

That's exactly what we did. We invited our friends, our family, and our fans to join us on the homestead. People came from all over the East Coast, which was cool. But what was even more special was that everyone brought their own homegrown goodies!

There was roasted turkey, fried chicken, and grass-fed beef hamburgers straight from the farm. There were salads like you wouldn't believe—leafy salads, cabbage salads, bean salads, berry salads, and fruit salads. All harvested right off the land. We had sweet corn on the cob with thick slabs of butter. We had mashed potatoes and sweet potatoes and fried potatoes and baked potatoes. And you know there were desserts of every size, shape, color, and flavor. But I'm going to resist describing them here because I don't want to make you any hungrier than you already are!

Even more than the food, I enjoyed being able to meet so many of the people who supported us in those early days by watching our videos and reading what I wrote. I loved the chance to look those folks in the eye, shake their hand, and express my gratitude for all the ways they had blessed me and my family.

Speaking of which, I do want to take a moment to say thank you for reading this book. (And thanks for making it all the way to the last chapter!) It has been a lot of work to put this together, but I've enjoyed the process of writing—and I hope very much you've enjoyed the process of reading.

In the end, though, you can read this book until you're bleary-eyed, but no homegrown tomatoes or eggs will ever come from it. To succeed in growing your own food you're going to have to take some very definite steps:

1. *Start growing.* Just get out there and plant! Start growing something— anything from a little pot of Bus Basil all the way to Crop Gardens and chickens. All of it is possible for you, but nothing will happen until you start.

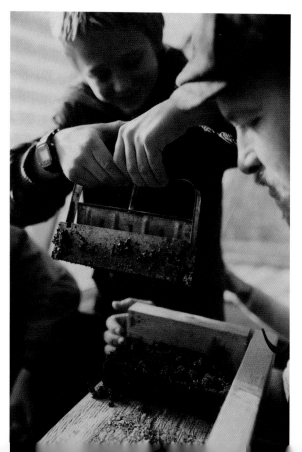
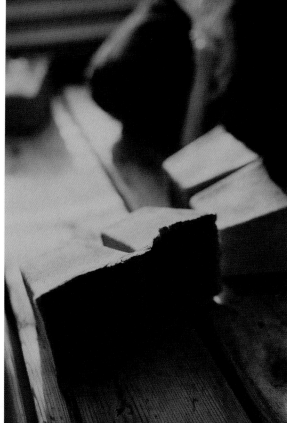

2. *Continue growing.* In some ways, getting started is the easy part. The next step is to keep going! Don't give up. Don't get discouraged. Keep the vision of abundance in front of you and let that drive you to continue the journey when you get to those places where you feel like quitting.

3. *Deal with failure.* I've said it already, but it's worth repeating: You're going to make mistakes as you pursue a more rooted life. Certainly you're going to fail. You'll probably kill something, too, but all of that is okay. Why? Because you'll create way more life than you kill. You'll succeed way more often than you fail. The best thing you can do is learn from those mistakes and keep moving forward.

4. *Enjoy the ride!* If you can't have fun while you're cultivating health and wellness for your family, what's the point? Yes, there's going to be work involved. Sometimes a lot of work. But I really encourage you to seek out ways to enjoy yourself in this process. Remember, grow what you love to eat. Find people you enjoy spending time with and invite them to join you for the "chores" of life. Make it a point to have fun!

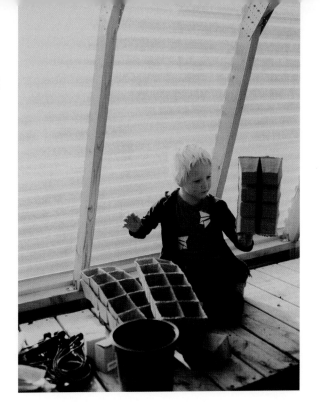

Recently I was on a live webinar when someone asked me for the top three things they could do to ensure success in homesteading. I loved this question because it was precise. There are dozens of things you can do to be successful at growing your own food—and I've tried to outline many of them in this book—but this question forced me to identify the cream of the crop. The best keys to success.

I think that's a great place to wind up this book. I can offer three keys to success that will help you maximize your efforts and investments in a more rooted way of life.

Stay Home (and Opt Out)

There's no easy way to say this, so I'll just spit it out: The number one key to success in the rooted life is for you to commit to being rooted. That means choosing to stay home as much as possible.

Like anything in life, if you want to achieve something great, you'll need to make sacrifices. Same thing with cultivating health and wellness. If you want to be rooted in a way that leads to true abundance for yourself and your family, you need to revolve your life around your home as much as possible—not the other way around.

Now, hopefully that sounds appealing to you. Given that you're reading this book, chances are good you're looking to escape a more hectic (and harmful) way of life, and you're ready to slow down a bit. That's great. Because that is the nature of the rooted life. Slow. Deliberate. Intentional. Giving rather than taking. Being rather than doing.

This reality increases the deeper you go

down the path. Growing your own food means you'll have gardens that need weeding and watering. You may have animals that need attention—sometimes lots of attention. Beyond the daily tasks, you'll need to be aware of what's going on within your home and around your home. That's what it means to be rooted.

Rebekah and I do everything we can from home. We work from home, we homeschool, we shop from home, we entertain from home. We even have home births! We don't go anywhere if we don't have to. Heck, we even found a mobile dog groomer and a chiropractor who makes house calls for our family. (Now all we have to do is figure out how to get our dentist to drive out this way, and we'll never have to leave.)

Choosing this lifestyle does mean we intentionally opt out of several typical elements in the "American Dream." Those include:

- *Sports and other extracurricular activities.* When you've got kids, nothing will pull you in different directions (and pull you away from home) like sports. We want our kids to get exercise and to socialize, of course, but we've found we can do that primarily at home. We take walks and fun runs, we hike our local mountain, we go swimming, and so on. We replace individual activities with family activities, and as a result we enjoy more time together.

- *Eating out.* This one was hard at first. Rebekah and I enjoyed our dating lives, which included a lot of dinner dates. But now that we've become so comfortable growing our own food, why would we go out to restaurants for the "privilege" of eating a meal that is way more expensive, way less healthy, and usually way less tasty than what we can produce ourselves?

- *Entertainment.* Same principle applies here. If there's something available that Rebekah and I can't experience at home—such as live theater or a concert—we'll occasionally bite the bullet and head to town. Otherwise, the good ol' internet keeps us plenty entertained at home.

- *Multiple cars.* We have just one car. It fits our whole family, and it's available whenever someone does need to get off the homestead for a while. We have no reason for two (or more) vehicles, which saves us money on car payments, gas, insurance, and maintenance.

Why do we choose to live this way? Because we love being home.

Yes, I know you need a social life. We do too. But being rooted means we go about it a little differently. First of all, when we want to spend time with people outside our family, we invite them to join us at our home. We like entertaining, so we choose to do it here.

And of course, choosing the rooted life doesn't mean *never* leaving the house. Our family goes to town. But when we do, we make a whole day of it. We plan ahead so that we can do everything we want to do, get everything we need to get, and then be present when we return home—not rushing out for this errand or that. Also, we do take vacations, although it's difficult given the amount of animals and other life we manage. For us, that means hiring a trained farmhand we trust who can fill in while we're gone.

In general, though, we choose to stay home as much as we can. That means we're near our gardens and our animals so that we can tend them regularly and quickly correct any problems that pop up. More importantly, being home isn't just good for our farm—it's good for our souls.

Be Strategic

The second key to success for the rooted life is to be strategic in everything you do. That means following these steps whenever possible:

- Have a goal.
- Create a plan.
- Implement the plan.
- Rework the plan.

When I say "Have a goal," I mean be specific. *I want to grow my own food* is nice, but it's not specific. Instead, set goals that have precise targets for you to aim at. *I want to grow 50 percent of our family's produce,* for example. Or, *I want my family to have one chicken in our freezer for every week of the year.*

Your mind is powerful. So are your desires. A good goal will drive you toward success, but you also need to give yourself a route to follow. That's why you need to make a plan. As Antoine de Saint-Exupéry said, "A goal without a plan is just a wish." So, each time you want to try something new in the rooted life—a Winter Harvest Garden, for example, or creating an Instant Chicken Garden—you need to match that goal with a plan.

Then you need to get to work. Implement the plan. Make it happen. Of course, there will be mistakes. Things will go wrong. When that happens, don't freak out. Just take a deep breath, maybe enjoy a cup of tea, rework your plan to account for what you've learned, and start again.

That's what success looks like in the rooted life.

Create a Community

I know, I know. You're feeling confused because I said the first key to success in the rooted life is to stay home and opt out, but now I'm saying you need to seek out or create a community. Well, the truth is those two ideas are not mutually exclusive. Rebekah and I know this from experience.

By its very nature, the rooted life (including choosing to stay home as much as possible) can lead to loneliness, which is not good. Loneliness is not abundance or wellness, and it's not something you have to settle for if you choose to grow a lot of your own food. Instead, you can create the community you need.

Like most things in the rooted life, that starts at home. My wife is my best friend. My children are some of my closest companions. These are relationships we have cultivated

with as much care as we cultivate our crops. (More, actually.) So, as I've been saying throughout these recent chapters, make an active, intentional effort to involve your family as much as possible in your efforts to grow your own food. Trust me, that investment will produce an incredible harvest.

Next, be alert for other people in your area who are doing what you want to do. Namely, growing their own food. If you see people with gardens or chickens or low tunnels or other indicators that they are pursuing the rooted life, turn into their driveway and say hello. Talk some shop. Ask questions about how they handle this problem or that problem. You just might forge a bond with some kindred spirits.

Of course, the internet is also a great resource for community. When we started documenting our lifestyle on YouTube, we

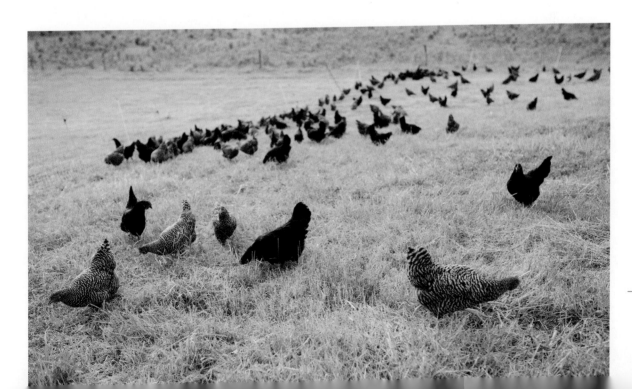

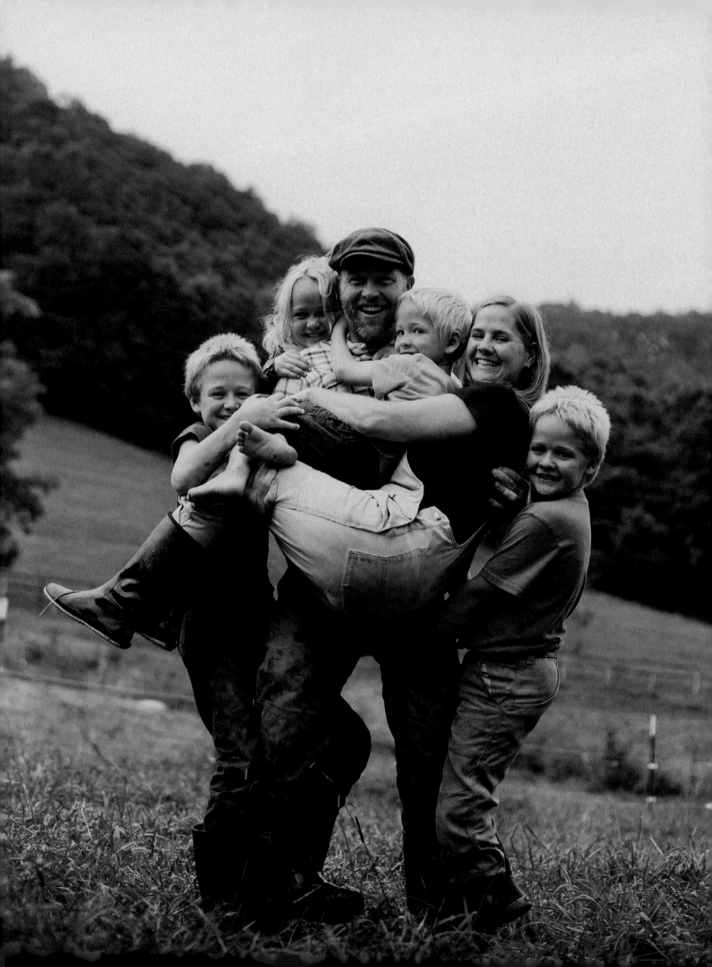

quickly amassed a following. Turns out others were feeling lonely, just like us, so reaching out to us helped them feel less isolated—and vice versa. Folks found us, emailed, then visited, and many became fast friends. One of our employees told us once that we're the most socialized homebodies she knows!

My point is that you can find community and still be rooted to your home. You just have to go about things a little differently.

Now It's Your Turn

What else can I say? Rebekah and I have done our best to share our story with you throughout these pages because our lives are rich. Our home is sweet. Each day is filled with laughter, adventure, and purpose. Oh, and good healthy food!

We want the same for you.

I don't know what has attracted you into considering the rooted life. Maybe it's saving money. Maybe it's health. Maybe it's the image of laughing children running through an abundant garden—or maybe the image of those same children working hard and building character out there among the chickens and the cows and the crops ready for harvest.

Let me say now that those dreams are good. But they are just dreams. When you jump into the rooted life, you'll find a reality that is way different than you ever expected— way more work and trouble, yes, but also way more joy. Way more *life*!

I truly believe that once you push through enough trials and begin to see this way of life for what it really is, you'll quickly become happier and more satisfied than you imagined possible. Sure, you might lose half of your green beans because you waited too long to harvest. You might have a meat chicken or two snatched up by an aerial predator. A rogue mole might sneak a few of your potatoes right out from under your nose. Those things happen.

But here's what else happens: You'll sit down to a meal that you not only cooked, but *grew*. You'll bless your family with roasted chicken, seasoned green beans, and mashed potatoes that all have a story—a story in which each of you had a place. A part. A connection.

You'll sit down together at that meal and think, *We grew this!* Yes, it will taste great. And yes, it will be much healthier and cheaper than what you ate in the past. But your joy will go deeper than all that. The experience will be special because you overcame obstacles and worked hard. Because you made it happen.

That's the real happy ending of the rooted life. The one you could never have imagined until you actually got out there and lived it.

So get out there and live it. Just plant!

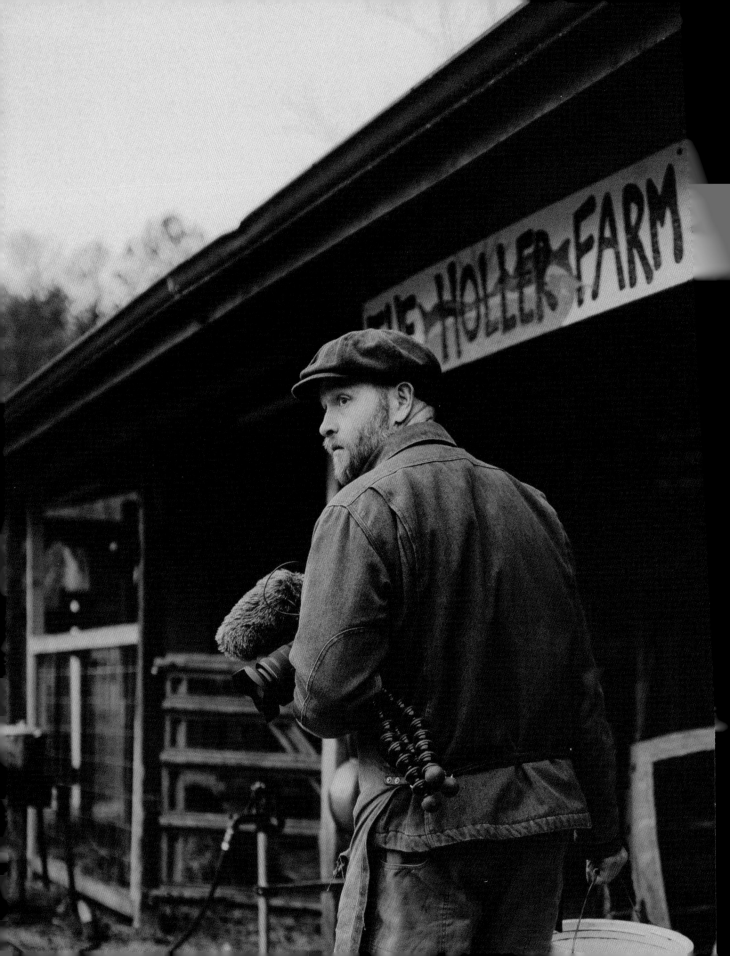

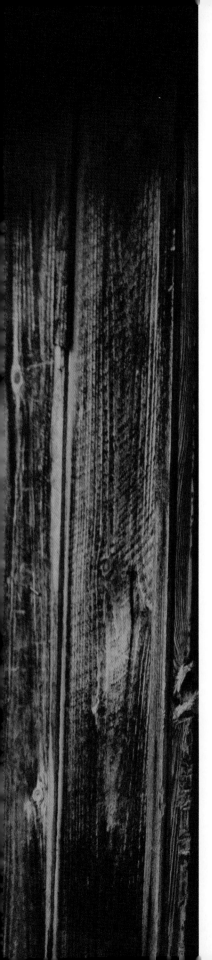

ACKNOWLEDGMENTS

True story: We were hanging out at a gathering talking about something food related when Rebekah said, "We ought to get some chickens." Unbelievably, someone walked by not five minutes later and asked if any of us wanted chickens. Uh, yes! Thank you, Don and Heidi Hendrix, for our very first posse. Unfortunately, two of those four chickens immediately escaped, and we never saw them again. Thank you, Joel Salatin and Harvey Ussery, for your books that showed me the way.

If you're gonna have chickens, you gotta have a garden. So thank you, John Roach, for installing our first veggie patch. We did well but made mucho mistakes. Thanks to Eliot Coleman's books, for giving me a system to follow.

Thank you, Lyme disease, for destroying my health and energy. If you hadn't forced me to quit market farming and slow down my homestead, I wouldn't have found a better way through Permaculture design. Thank you, Ethan Hardin, for volunteering every week to keep my homestead alive during those dark days.

Thank you, Steve Meeks, for being a mentor to me and handing me *The 4-Hour Workweek*. Thank you, more importantly, for cheering for me all along the way. I couldn't market farm anymore but still wanted to be in the food-growing movement. That book interested me, because four hours was all the time I felt I had, and it opened up the world of internet business. I used those concepts to launch my first learning product, *Permaculture Chickens*. Interestingly enough, I wasn't going to be the star of that production—someone else was—but their publisher got in the way. That's when I somehow got the strength to tell Rebekah (even though I didn't feel capable), "Maybe I could be the star expert." To which she replied, "For sure." I'm forever indebted to you for ALWAYS believing in me! That means EVERYTHING to me.

Thank you, Cassie Langstraat, for being my very first customer (and eventually helping to convince me to monetize my YouTube channel). Speaking of the YouTube channel, I don't know if we ever would have vlogged had Sam (from the Sam and Nia YouTube channel) not found out she was pregnant and got a viral video. That's when we discovered vlogging,

and it turns out it was a perfect match for our family. A big ol' Uncle Justin hug (and thank you, thank you, thank you) to our faithful vlog fans and customers who have become our extended family.

It was actually a vlog fan who said I should write a book about my continuous (and hilarious) adventures trying to find Mr. Brown's shoes (my son). Thank you, Kathy, my agent, for taking me on as a debut author and advising that I write a nonfiction book first, then a

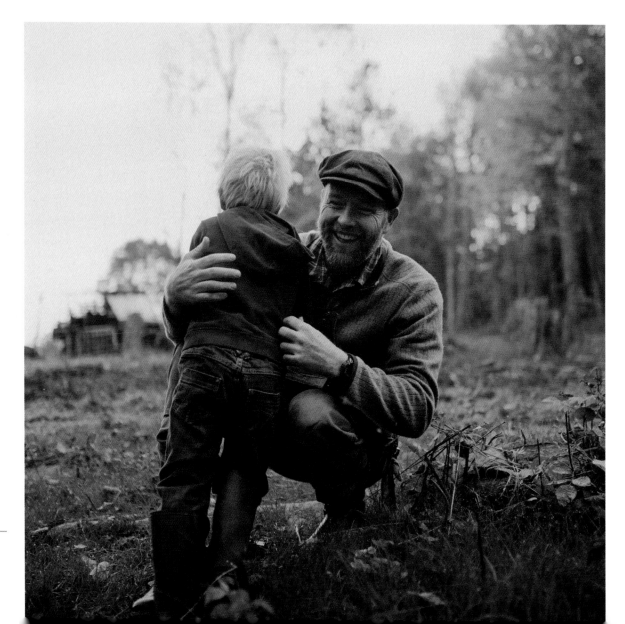

children's book. This has been a wonderful detour, and to tell you the truth, writing a nonfiction book has always been a dream of mine.

Oh my word, Daisy, my contact at Hachette. Thank you so much for believing in me and offering me such a generous deal. You won't be disappointed! Furthermore, this book wouldn't be so full of lifestyle content had you not kept steering us in that direction. Turns out the lifestyle stuff is my happy place and will likely be the work that outlasts me. Please tell your husband he did a most excellent job thinking of the title! Oh, and you introduced me to Sam O'Neal right when I needed him the most. I had written the manuscript, but we all felt it lacked structure and connection. If I'm Frodo in *The Lord of the Rings*, Sam is my Sam. The world would know something was missing in this book without your contribution, Sam. It certainly helped that you're also a big fan of *Nacho Libre* and we could laugh together at the various references throughout the script. Best of all you respected me for the final say. Like that time you removed the part where I get "lucky," then you put it back when I called you on it. That, my friend, earned you my trust, and definitely earned you more work from me. That reminds me, I need to send you that children's book manuscript. Check your email!

Then, of course, there's my chiddlers. Thank you so much for wanting to be with me. For being my companions. For helping me get stuff done. Thank you for dreaming and doing things "wrong" and showing me that sometimes there's a better way than what the textbooks say. Thank you for dwelling so much in my world of work and for inviting me into your world of play. We balance each other perfectly. Last, but certainly not least, please know that I'm proud of each and every one of you.

Finally, I must thank YOU, the reader, for buying this book. For trusting and believing in me so much that you would invest in such a resource. You've noticed I couldn't have done any of this alone (including homesteading). I needed guides for every step of the book writing and homestead journey. Books helped me early on, but I had to fill in a lot of gaps myself to apply what I was learning to the homestead. I'm honored to be such a guide for all you "crazy chicken ladies" out there. Call me "Uncle Justin" if you want to. After all, we're all a part of a bigger family working together to make the world a better place for our grandchildren.

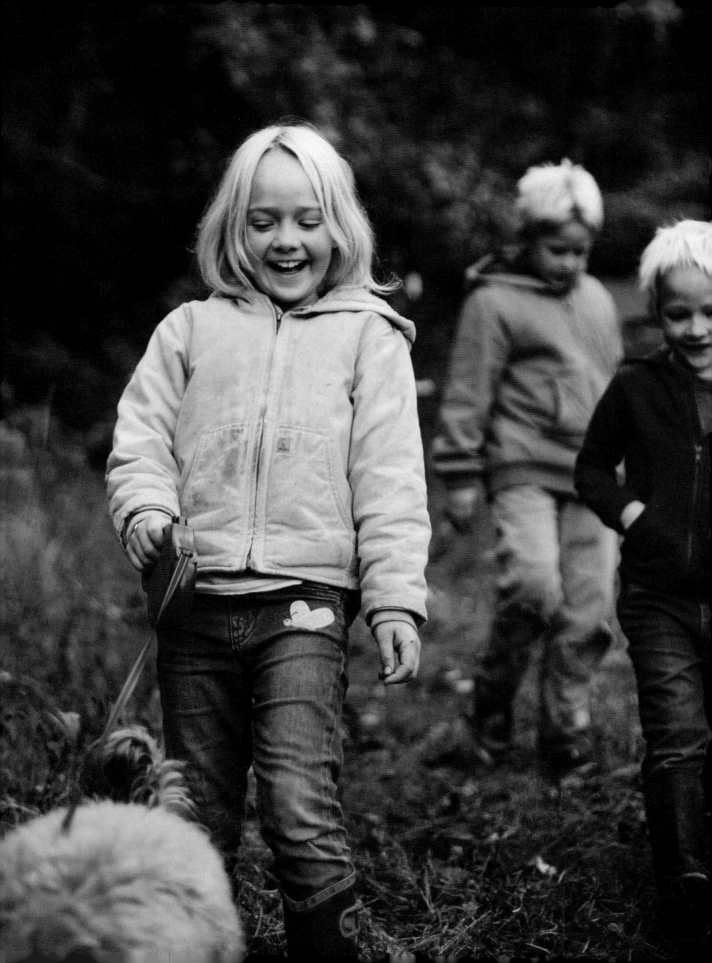

RESOURCES

There's lots of great information available out there when it comes to growing your own food. Here are some of the sources Rebekah and I have created ourselves, plus some by others we trust.

Websites

TheRootedLife.com. This is a free website that we have put together specifically to complement this book. Here you will find many detailed plans and supply lists for the systems we describe in these pages. We will keep this updated, so make sure to check back often.

YouTube.com/JustinRhodesVlog. Our YouTube channel! You'll find tons of videos here with helpful instructions, step-by-step guides, and plenty of hilarious and heartwarming windows into our family and our farm.

AbundancePlus.com. This is our streaming site and app. When you're ready to seriously dive into growing your own food, this is where you can find more entertainment, community, and know-how to help you along the way.

Books

Eliot Coleman, *Four-Season Harvest* (Winter Harvest Garden)

Eliot Coleman, *The New Organic Grower* (Crop Garden)

Napoleon Hill, *Think and Grow Rich* (encourages the abundance mindset)

Bill Mollison, *Introduction to Permaculture* (essential design principles)

Joel Salatin, *Pastured Poultry Profits* (raising chickens for profit)

Joel Salatin, *Polyface Micro* (farm scale management)

Harvey Ussery, *The Small-Scale Poultry Flock* (raising chickens)

Carrie Vitt, *The Grain-Free Family Table* (cookbook)

Danielle Walker, *Celebrations* (cookbook)

Danielle Walker, *Eat What You Love* (cookbook)

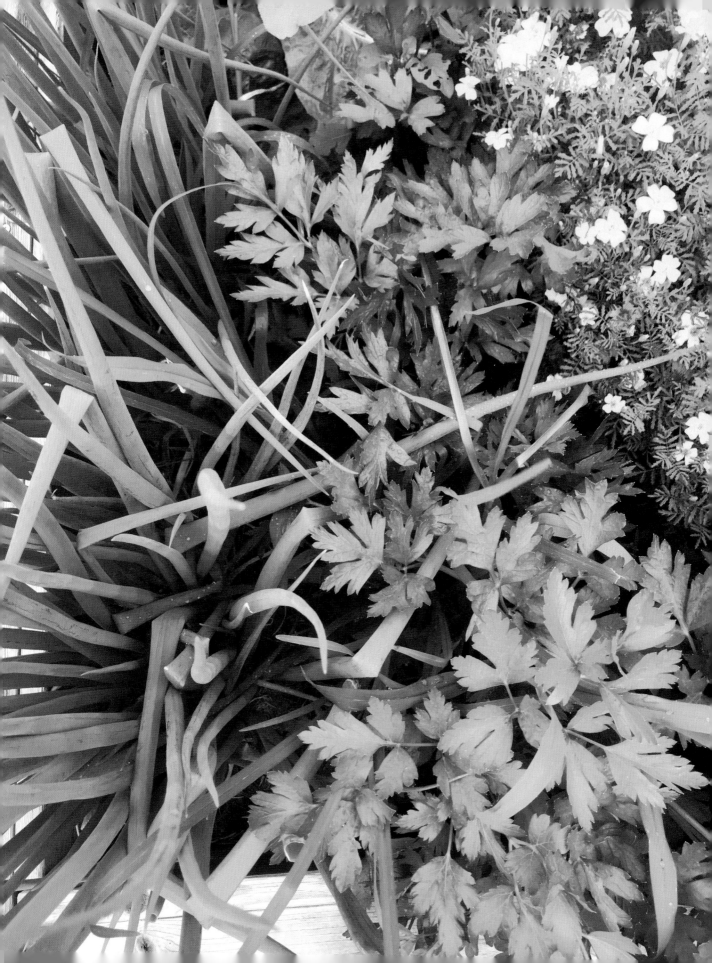

APPENDIX

Best Homestead Elements

Element	Setup Time	Harvesttime	Weekly Chore Time	Cost	Chore Difficulty	Space	Yield
Container Garden	15 minutes	10 minutes per season	5 minutes	$	Very easy	Size of the containers	Several plants per container
Herb Garden	15 minutes	10 minutes per season	5 minutes	$	Very easy	Size of the containers	50–100 percent of culinary herbs each year
Bulletproof Garden	2–4 hours	1 hour per season	15 minutes	$	Easy	4 x 8 feet	25 percent of a family's veggies during the growing season
Raised Beds	4–8 hours	1–2 hours per season	15 minutes	$$$	Easy	4 x 8 feet	25 percent of veggies during the growing season
Crop Garden	1 day	2 hours per season	1 hour	$$	Moderate	24 x 50 feet	50–75 percent of veggies during the growing season
Chicken Tractor	4 hours	1 minute daily	1 hour	$$	Easy	3 x 8 feet	3–4 chickens, 45–52 dozen eggs each year
Instant Chicken Garden	4 hours	1–2 hours per season	15 minutes	$$	Easy	4 x 8 feet	25 percent of veggie needs during the growing season
Compost Corner	4 hours	1 minute daily	1 hour	$$	Moderate	You choose the size of your run, but at least 3 square feet per bird	3–4 chickens, 45–52 dozen eggs each year

Garden Spacing Guide

Spacing for Herbs

Herbs	Basil	Cilantro	Dill	Oregano	Parsley	Sage	Rosemary	Thyme
Plants / square foot	3-4	6	1	1	4	1	1	3-4

Spacing for a Bulletproof Garden

Crops	Lettuces	Kale	Swiss Chard	Collards	Spinach	Tomatoes	Peppers	Broccoli
Plants / square foot	3-4	3-4	3-4	3-4	6	1	1	1

Crops	Cabbages	Yellow Squashes	Zucchini	Pumpkins	Cucumbers	Watermelons	Cantaloupes
Plants / square foot	1	1	1	1	½	½	½

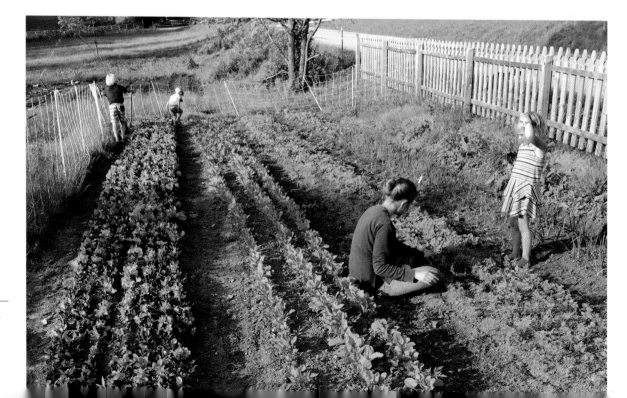

Spacing for a Crop Garden

Note: A garden "bed" is 30 inches wide by 50 feet long.

Crops	Number of rows per bed	Spacing within each row	Number of plants per bed	Number of seeds per block	Number of blocks per foot in each bed
Lettuces	3	6 inches	300	1	6
Kale	3	6 inches	300	1	6
Swiss Chard	3	6 inches	300	1	6
Broccoli	2	2 feet	50	1	1
Cabbages	2	1 foot	100	1	2
Tomatoes	1	18 inches	33	N/A	N/A
Peppers	1	1 foot	50	N/A	N/A
Carrots	4	2 inches	1,200	N/A	N/A
Cucumbers	1	12 inches	50	N/A	N/A
Corn	2	6 inches	200	N/A	N/A
Spaghetti Squashes	1	2 feet	25	N/A	N/A
Yellow Squashes	1	2 feet	25	N/A	N/A
Acorn Squashes	1	2 feet	25	N/A	N/A
Zucchini	1	2 feet	25	N/A	N/A
Pumpkins	1	2 feet	25	N/A	N/A
Cantaloupes	1	5 feet	10	N/A	N/A
Watermelons	1	5 feet	10	N/A	N/A

Spacing for a Winter Harvest Garden

Note: A garden "bed" is 30 inches wide by 50 feet long.

Crops	Number of rows per bed	Spacing within each row	Number of plants per bed	Number of seeds per block	Number of blocks per foot in each bed
Beets	2	4 inches	300	4	6
Carrots	4	2 inches	1,200	N/A	N/A
Turnips	2	2 inches	300	4	6
Broccoli	2	2 feet	50	1	1
Brussels Sprouts	2	2 feet	50	1	1
Cabbages	2	1 foot	100	1	2
Swiss Chard	3	6 inches	300	1	6
Collards	3	6 inches	300	1	6
Kale	3	6 inches	300	1	6
Lettuces	3	6 inches	300	1	6
Spinach	3	3 inches	600	1	12

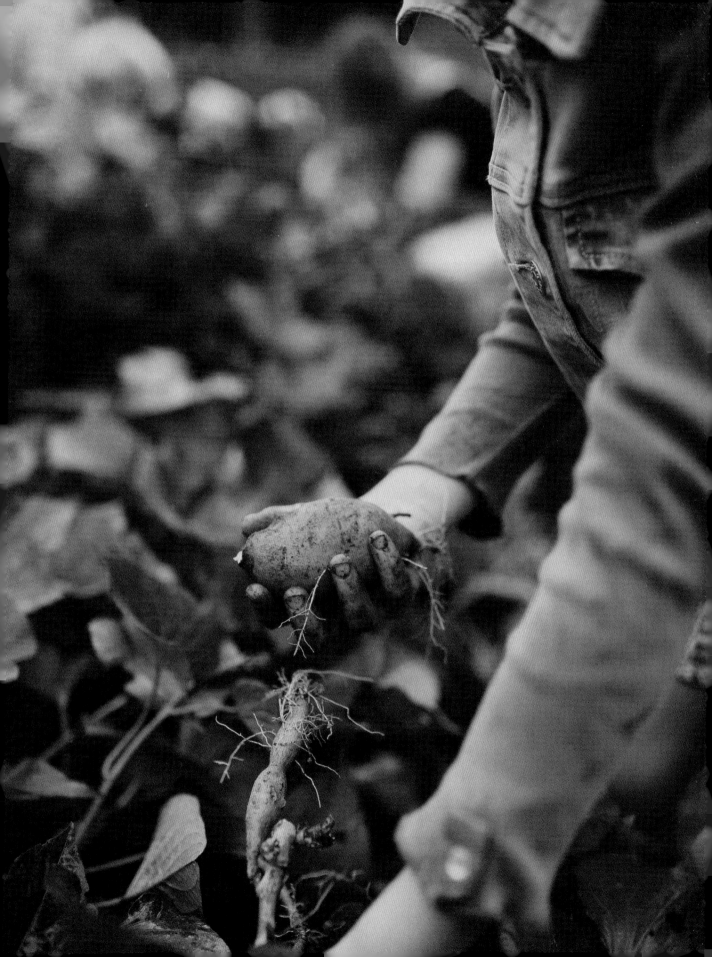

ABOUT THE AUTHOR

JUSTIN AND REBEKAH RHODES are film producers and authors, teaching folks to work with nature to produce their own sustenance and live a more abundant life. Seasoned homesteaders, the Rhodeses have enjoyed many years of practicing "beyond organic" and Permaculture methods on their 75-acre family farm near Asheville, North Carolina. Justin trained under the highly accredited Geoff Lawton of PRI Australia for his Permaculture Design Certificate (PDC) and maintains a close mentoring relationship with Joel Salatin of Polyface Farm.

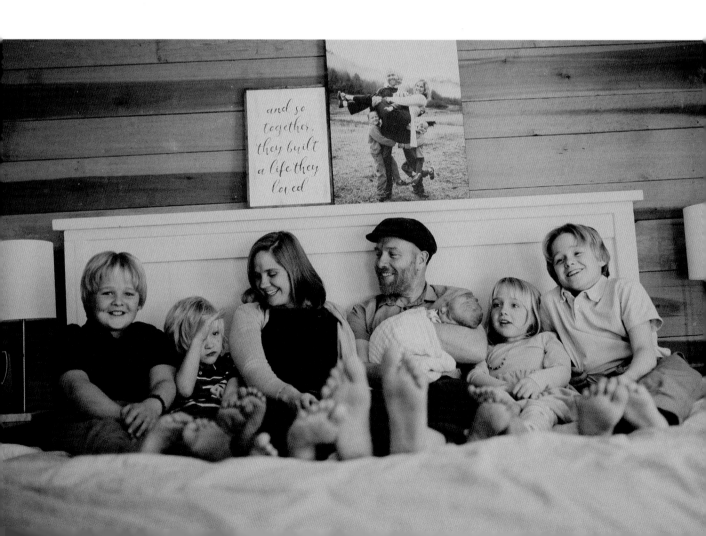